THERAPEUTIC COMMUNICATIONS FOR HEALTH CARE

THIRD EDITION

CAROL D. TAMPARO
AND
WILBURTA Q. LINDH

THERAPEUTIC COMMUNICATIONS FOR HEALTH CARE

THIRD EDITION

CAROL D. TAMPARO

BS, PhD, CMA-A
Former Dean of Business and Allied Health
Lake Washington Technical College
Kirkland, Washington

WILBURTA Q. LINDH

CMA
Professor Emerita
Highline Community College
Des Moines, Washington

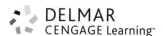
DELMAR
CENGAGE Learning

Australia • Brazil • Canada • Mexico • Singapore • Spain • United Kingdom • United States

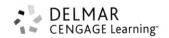
DELMAR
CENGAGE Learning™

**Therapeutic Communications
for Health Care, Third Edition**

Carol D. Tamparo,
Wilburta Q. Lindh

Vice President, Health Care
  Business Unit: William Brottmiller

Director of Learning Solutions:
  Matthew Kane

Managing Editor: Marah Bellegarde

Acquisitions Editor:
  Matthew Seeley

Product Manager:
  Jadin Babin-Kavanaugh

Editorial Assistant: Nicole Bruno

Marketing Director:
  Jennifer McAvey

Marketing Manager:
  Michele McTighe

Marketing Coordinator:
  Andrea Eobstel

Technology Director: Laurie Davis

Technology Project Managers:
  Mary Colleen Liburdi

Production Director: Carolyn Miller

Content Project Manager:
  Anne Sherman

Art Director: Jack Pendleton

For product information and technology assistance, contact us at
Cengage Learning Customer & Sales Support, 1-800-354-9706

For permission to use material from this text or product,
submit all requests online at **www.cengage.com/permissions**
Further permissions questions can be emailed to
permissionrequest@cengage.com

ExamView® and ExamView Pro® are registered trademarks of FSCreations, Inc. Windows is a registered trademark of the Microsoft Corporation used herein under license. Macintosh and Power Macintosh are registered trademarks of Apple Computer, Inc. Used herein under license.

© 2007 Cengage Learning. All Rights Reserved. Cengage Learning WebTutor™ is a trademark of Cengage Learning.

Library of Congress Control Number: 2007021531

ISBN-13: 978-1-4180-3264-7

ISBN-10: 1-4180-3264-6

Delmar
Executive Woods
5 Maxwell Drive
Clifton Park, NY 12065
USA

Cengage Learning is a leading provider of customized learning solutions with office locations around the globe, including Singapore, the United Kingdom, Australia, Mexico, Brazil, and Japan. Locate your local office at
www.cengage.com/global

Cengage Learning products are represented in Canada by Nelson Education, Ltd.

To learn more about Delmar, visit **www.cengage.com/delmar**

Purchase any of our products at your local bookstore or at our preferred online store
www.ichapters.com

Printed in the United States of America
6 7 11

DEDICATION

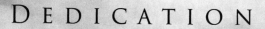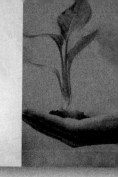

This book is dedicated to every instructor, professor, student, or health care professional who recognizes and practices the all-important component of comprehensive health care—therapeutic communication.

CONTENTS

CHAPTER 2

MULTICULTURAL THERAPEUTIC COMMUNICATION 28

CHAPTER 3

THE HELPING INTERVIEW 56

CHAPTER 5

THE THERAPEUTIC RESPONSE TO STRESSED AND ANXIOUS CLIENTS 102

CHAPTER 6

THE THERAPEUTIC RESPONSE TO FEARFUL, ANGRY, AGGRESSIVE, ABUSED, OR ABUSIVE CLIENTS 124

CHAPTER 7

THE THERAPEUTIC RESPONSE TO DEPRESSED AND/OR SUICIDAL CLIENTS 154

CHAPTER 8

THE THERAPEUTIC RESPONSE TO CLIENTS WITH SUBSTANCE USE DISORDERS 176

CHAPTER 9

THE THERAPEUTIC RESPONSE TO CLIENTS WITH LIFE-ALTERING ILLNESS   192

CHAPTER 10

THE THERAPEUTIC RESPONSE TO CLIENTS EXPERIENCING LOSS, GRIEF, DYING, AND DEATH   208

APPENDIX A

THEORIES OF HUMAN GROWTH AND DEVELOPMENT 224

APPENDIX B

PREFACE

Therapeutic Communications for Health Care is a critical and key component of health care for any client. Today's climate of health care is both technical and clinical. Because interaction with clients and patients can often be rushed, the client may be left feeling devalued and with many unanswered questions. This text addresses the critical need in health care today for successful therapeutic communication between health care staff and clients. Effective communication with patients can decrease stress, increase patient compliance, and result in a positive experience for all involved. Members of all health care professions will benefit from the information in this text, including students of allied health programs and nursing programs.

Instructors at all levels of health care indicate that teaching "soft skills" like good communication is one of the most difficult tasks they face in the classroom. Students in all areas of health care can be taught the clinical and technical skills with the right amount of instructional oversight and practice; teaching students how to respond therapeutically in all situations is more difficult to teach in a classroom setting.

ABOUT THIS TEXT

The key to learning the soft skills is exposure and the ability to think critically in the moment. This text introduces the reader to the purpose and reality of therapeutic communication in all types of settings, including how to communicate with multicultural clients, clients of varying ages, circumstances, and stages of illness, as well as health care peers and professionals. The reader will learn how to respond therapeutically to clients who are stressed, anxious, fearful, angry, aggressive, abused or abusive, and depressed or suicidal. Special attention is given to clients with substance use disorders or life-altering illnesses, and to clients experiencing loss, grief, dying, or death.

Features

- Each chapter opens with a case study that puts chapter content into a real-world context, to provide a framework for learning.

- Sections focus in on the therapeutic response to health care client situations, applying techniques discussed to specific situations and special patient needs in health care.

- Both good and bad examples of communication are given, with a discussion of what could have been said or done to make the communication more therapeutic.

- Icons highlight and organize important information for users.

- End-of-chapter exercises, numerous case studies, and critical thinking exercises in each chapter assist the user with comprehension and self-assessment.

New to This Edition

- Chapter 2 now contains comprehensive information on the topic of multicultural therapeutic communication, filled with helpful examples and suggestions.

- *Stop and Consider* and *For Further Consideration* features invite students to think critically about chapter content as they read, and provide opportunity for in-class discussions and thinking beyond the chapter.

- Icons highlight important *Legal, Cultural, Growth & Development*, and *Self-Awareness* topics.

- Illustrations have been provided by Benjamin Towle to enhance the subject matter.

- Appendices provide a review of important information on theories of human growth and development, as well as a description of common defense mechanisms; both appendices feature exercises for extra practice.

- Free StudyWARE CD-ROM features additional chapter quizzes for self-test and review, as well as 20 case scenarios with video clips and critical thinking questions.

HOW TO USE THIS TEXT

The third edition of *Therapeutic Communications for Health Care* is designed to make the learning process as intuitive as possible. Here is a brief description of each feature and its intended use.

Chapter Objectives

Chapter Objectives may be used to test your knowledge of the key facts presented in the chapter. Use these objectives, together with review and *For Further Consideration* questions and exercises to test your understanding of the chapter's content.

Opening Case Study

The "real-world" case studies introduced within each chapter serve as a springboard for discussion, provide food for thought, and can be a means to emphasize key points in the chapter. Through these case studies you will come to understand some of the stimulating challenges faced by health care professionals and gain insight into how these challenges are overcome.

Key Terms

All key terms appear in bold at the first occurrence for easy identification. The glossary provides definitions for all key terms.

Stop and Consider

The *Stop and Consider* feature occurs throughout the learning process and provides an opportunity for critical thinking discussions as you learn.

Icons

Icons for *Self-Awareness, Culture, Legal,* and *Growth & Development* information are interspersed throughout the chapters and highlight important topic reminders.

The Therapeutic Response

This feature applies techniques discussed within the chapter to specific topics and age groups. Learners will achieve greater success with therapeutic communications in all situations with continued practice and evaluation of a therapeutic response.

Exercises

Exercises at the end of each chapter present interesting and interactive ways for learners to apply theory and skills presented in the chapter to specific environments and situations. These exercises are practical and help learners become confident in using new knowledge and skills. Points may be awarded for completed exercises as desired.

Multiple Choice Questions

These questions test the learner's comprehension of the chapter with structured multiple-choice questions.

For Further Consideration

This feature provides opportunities for learners to think beyond the text. Chapter material, as well as personal insight and judgment, will be required to respond.

Case Studies

The actual case studies challenge learners to think through options for solving problems critically. Often there is no one correct answer, nor should there be, and students will have to consider the consequences of their decisions and recommendations.

HOW TO USE THE STUDYWARE™ CD-ROM

The StudyWARE™ interactive software helps you learn and apply the concepts in *Therapeutic Communications for Health Care*. As you study each chapter in the text, be sure to explore the quizzes and case studies in the corresponding chapter in the software. Use StudyWARE™ as your own private tutor to help you learn the material in your *Therapeutic Communications for Health Care* textbook.

Getting started is easy. Install the software by inserting the CD-ROM into your computer's CD-ROM drive and following the on-screen instructions. When you open the software, enter your first and last name so the software can store your quiz results. Then choose a chapter from the menu to take a quiz or explore one of the case studies.

You can take the quizzes in both *Practice Mode* and *Quiz Mode*. Use Practice Mode to improve your mastery of the material. You have multiple tries to get the answers correct. Instant feedback tells you whether you're right or wrong—and helps you learn quickly by explaining why an answer was correct or incorrect. Use Quiz Mode when you are ready to test yourself and keep a record of your scores.

Review the case studies and answer the questions that follow to enhance your critical thinking in the StudyWARE abilities. Each case contains either a video clip or an image to bring the case to life. You can either print your responses for the instructor, or check your answers against the expert answers.

INSTRUCTOR SUPPLEMENTS

The following supplements are available for instructors to enhance the use of *Therapeutic Communications for Health Care* in the classroom:

Online Companion, ISBN 1-4180-3265-4

The *Online Companion* contains password-protected instructor resources such as an Instructor's Manual, Computerized Test Bank, and Power-Point™ presentation for instructors. For access to the Online Companion site, contact your Delmar Sales Representative, or go to http://www.delmarlearning.com/companions/ for more information.

Instructor's Manual

The Online Companion site features an electronic *Instructor's Manual* that is packed with everything an instructor needs to be effective and efficient in the classroom. The Instructor's Manual includes complete answer keys to textbook questions, as well as expert answers to the case studies in the book and on the StudyWARE™ CD-ROM. It also includes complete lesson plans with suggested media and other visual aids, a complete presentation topic-by-topic outline, and a discussion of how to use the textbook features and supplements to your advantage in the classroom.

Computerized Test Bank and PowerPoint™ Presentation

Also included at the Online Companion site is a *Computerized Test Bank*, featuring over 350 customizable test questions, including true/false, multiple choice, and short answer question types. A 250-slide PowerPoint™ presentation based on the textbook is also available at the site.

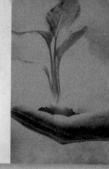

ACKNOWLEDGMENTS
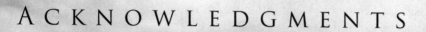

The authors and the publisher would like to thank the following reviewers for their invaluable feedback:

Patricia Bortnem, BSN, M.Ed.
Allied Health Instructor
Southeast Technical Institute
Brookings, South Dakota

Diana Dechichio, RN, BSN, M.Ed.
Instructor, Associate Degree program
Coastal Education Institute
Tampa, Florida

Mary Ann Edelman, MS, CNS, RN
Assistant Professor of Nursing
Kingsborough Community College
Brooklyn, New York

Mary Gormandy White, MA
Director/Co-Owner
Mobile Technical Institute
Mobile, Alabama

Claire E. Maday-Travis MA, MBA, CPHQ
Director of Allied Health Programs
The Salter School
Worcester, Massachusetts
   and
Lead Evening/Weekend Administrator
Quinsigamond Community College
Worcester, Massachusetts

Dana McNeeley, RN, MSN
Assistant Professor of Nursing
Lansing School of Nursing and Health Sciences
Bellarmine University
Louisville, Kentucky

Jean Mousseau, M.Ed., OTR/L
Assistant Professor—Department of Nursing
Manatee Community College
Bradenton, Florida

Charmaine Parker, LPN
Medical Assisting Program Director
Wake Technical Community College
Raleigh, North Carolina

Patricia A. Rahe, MSN, BSN, RN
Professor, General Education and Support Services
Ivy Tech Community College of Indiana, Lawrenceburg Campus
Lawrenceburg, Indiana

Connie Rockstad, RN, MSN
Director of Nursing
Whatcom Community College
Bellingham, Washington

About the Authors

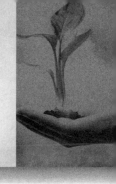

Carol D. Tamparo and Wilburta (Billie) Q. Lindh are co-authors of numerous health-related texts used by medical assistants and allied health care professionals throughout the United States. Both are Certified Medical Assistants with more than 25 years of experience in the field and in higher education. The authors have combined education and experience at the community college, four-year university, and graduate school levels. Their goal as educators was always to teach and model successful therapeutic communication in health care, and they continue to pursue this goal as authors.

Avenue for Feedback

Authors can be contacted at

Carol D. Tamparo, ctamparo@comcast.net
Wilburta Q. Lindh, billie.q.l@comcast.net

Therapeutic Communications for Health Care

Third Edition

Carol D. Tamparo

and

Wilburta Q. Lindh

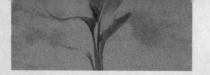

CHAPTER
1

THERAPEUTIC COMMUNICATION

CHAPTER OBJECTIVES

The learner should strive to meet the following chapter objectives and demonstrate an understanding of the facts and principles presented in this chapter through written and oral communication.

- Define key terms as presented in the glossary.
- List at least two characteristics of human and technical relations skills.
- Compare/contrast social and therapeutic communications.
- Describe at least five influences on perception.
- Discuss *self-awareness*.
- Differentiate between the *ideal self*, the *public self*, and the *real self*.
- List at least six questions to ask before entering a helping profession.
- List and define the four basic elements of the communication cycle.
- Identify the four modes or channels of communication most pertinent in our everyday exchanges.
- Analyze the five Cs of communication and describe their effectiveness.
- Identify and explain the two keys to successful communication.
- Demonstrate nonverbal communication behaviors.
- Identify three listening goals for the health care professional.

- Discuss the influence of technology on communication.
- Describe a minimum of six roadblocks to communication.

OPENING CASE STUDY

An elderly woman, Mrs. Nelson, was attacked by a German shepherd while walking her toy poodle. The German shepherd came out from his yard, attacking Mrs. Nelson and her poodle on the sidewalk. Serious injuries resulted.

Mrs. Nelson was pushed onto the pavement, falling backward and striking her head. A deep, 5-inch laceration was made in the back of the skull, and heavy bleeding resulted. There were two puncture wounds in her ring finger from the dog's bite. The finger was fractured in two places. In the emergency room, she learned she also had a fractured coccyx. The toy poodle, also seriously injured, later survived emergency surgery at a veterinary clinic.

Mrs. Nelson was treated with care and compassion in an overcrowded emergency room on a Sunday night. Many health care professionals were involved in her care. Several efforts failed to stop the bleeding from the head wound, and it was several hours before Mrs. Nelson was released to go home with her finger in a splint, her head wound sutured, and a very tight bandage around her head.

She was advised to see her personal physician the next morning for a blood test and to return in three days either to the emergency room or to her physician to have the stitches removed.

Her family called and took her to her personal physician the next morning, with her emergency room records in hand.

STOP AND CONSIDER

You are the office assistant. What will you say to Mrs. Nelson when she arrives? What will you do for Mrs. Nelson?

The medical assistant told Mrs. Nelson she would have to wait because the doctor did not see patients without prior appointments. Mrs. Nelson explained that the emergency room physician said it was important the test be run in the morning. After more than an hour, her personal physician agreed to see her and perform the blood test.

The physician hurriedly checked the head wound and the finger, and asked the assistant to redress the wound. Mrs. Nelson's hair was badly matted with dried blood, and the assistant was uneasy about touching it. However, she replaced the bandage and released her with no instructions to return. The bandage was so loose that it fell off in the afternoon.

STOP AND CONSIDER

1. What might Mrs. Nelson's feelings be right now?
2. Identify the positive actions in this case study.
3. Identify the negative actions in this case study.

Mrs. Nelson had hoped that her personal physician would be able to discuss her fears and anxieties, answer her questions, and give her some assurances about recovery. Mrs. Nelson's emotional needs were greater than her need for technical medical care. (See Maslow in Appendix A.) When it was time to have the stitches removed, she returned to the hospital, where she had been treated with care and concern.

She was embarrassed about the dried blood in her hair, still present due to the instructions not to get the wound wet, so the assistant who helped the physician remove the stitches used a warm wash cloth and peroxide to gently remove most of the dried blood. The physician told her the head and finger wounds were healing nicely, but that the coccyx fracture would cause her discomfort for quite some time. Mrs. Nelson left the hospital a little less traumatized, knowing it would be several weeks before she would feel like herself again.

Three months later, Mrs. Nelson needed a physician's summary of her recovery process and any expected complications for insurance purposes. She returned to her primary care physician, who said, "There is nothing I can do for you now. Your head wound has healed nicely. You saw the orthopedic surgeon about your finger. I have no idea how long you will have pain from the coccyx fracture, and neither would any other physician."

Still uncomfortable about her physician's response, she chose to see another physician. In her interview with the new physician, the verbal exchange turned to the accident. The physician leaned forward, seeking out the cause of Mrs. Nelson's concern, and said, "Gosh, tell me what happened." In less than five minutes, she poured out her story.

Recognizing Mrs. Nelson's needs, the physician asked, "How is your dog?" He also commented, "It certainly seems to me that you should be able to safely walk your dog on a public sidewalk." He then proceeded to examine her.

Technically, this physician could do no more for the woman than either her primary care physician or the emergency room physician. What this physician did do is listen to her, acknowledge her trauma, verify that she was not at fault, and assure her that any medical needs would be cared for to the best of his ability.

INTRODUCTION

This case study describes an actual ordeal, and illustrates both positive and negative communication and human relations skills. In this chapter, you will become more aware of how your personal perceptions affect your communication style. You will be introduced to basic communication and listening skills to help you respond therapeutically to the needs of your clients.

HUMAN AND TECHNICAL RELATIONS SKILLS

Human relations skills, sometimes referred to as interpersonal skills, are employed in both personal and professional relationships. Some situations will be pleasant and fun; others will be unpleasant, strained, and unsatisfactory. Human relations skills include verbal and nonverbal communications, how you communicate and whether you are aware of the effect you have on others, and the language used.

An example of human relations skills from this scenario is the care and compassionate treatment Mrs. Nelson received at the emergency room, as contrasted with the irritation about the disruption to the schedule and the impersonal treatment she received from the physician's office personnel.

Technical skills represent those specialized skills that are required to deliver and support professional medical care. The preceding scenario illustrates several technical skills demonstrated by the staff in the emergency room, the lab and X-ray staff support, and the assistant who bandaged the wounds. The physicians who assessed the injuries and followed appropriate medical-care guidelines exhibited technical skills.

In the health care setting, neither human relations skills nor technical skills are sufficient by themselves. You must have a combination of the two.

SOCIAL AND THERAPEUTIC PROFESSIONAL COMMUNICATIONS

Human relations skills are translated into social and therapeutic communications when there is contact with persons seeking attention. Social communication requires nonspecific professional skills. For instance, you may offer assistance to an elderly gentleman removing his coat in the office, or you may dry the tears of a child who has just had an injection.

Therapeutic professional communication requires specific, well-defined professional skills. When you instruct a client regarding preparation for a flexible sigmoidoscopy, or when you explain the billing procedures to a new client, specific, well-defined professional skills are being used.

Therapeutic professional communication takes place between a person who has a specific need and a person who is skilled in techniques that can alleviate or diminish that problem. As in human relations skills, however, how you feel about yourself can directly affect how successful you are in social and therapeutic communications.

INFLUENCES ON LIFE

A number of influences greatly impact our lives and dominate how we feel about ourselves and how we feel others perceive us. A few of these influences are listed.

Genetic Influences

Inherited traits, such as height, body structure, and skin color, are defined and established by the genes passed on during fertilization. Even our gender influences perception.

Cultural Influences

Every culture has its own customs and traditions that directly influence the person we are and how we are perceived. For example, in Western medical tradition, we look directly at someone when speaking and often address individuals using first names. In many cultures, however, it is disrespectful to look directly at another person (especially one in authority), or to use first names when addressing them. This topic is discussed more fully in Chapter 2, "Multicultural Therapeutic Communication."

Economic Influences

A family's financial status relates directly to the type of education and life experiences they possess. If you were born and raised in poverty, your perception of life and others is likely to be much different than if you were born and raised in affluence. The amount and type of education and job-training experience is a direct influence on perception.

Life Experiences

Life experiences are great teachers. Those who have experienced grief and loss react differently from those who have not. Whether life's trials have been fairly easy or very harsh will influence one's lifestyle.

Spiritual and Moral Values

Spiritual beliefs influence perception. A spiritual belief in one's life can influence an individual's attitude when caring for other's needs. Spirituality generally encourages a reach beyond self to guide and care for others. Values or morals, the rules we live by or habits of conduct, are important in relation to self and others.

Models/Mentors

Models are found in national leaders, parents, teachers, spiritual guides, and public figures. They can be either positive or negative, but are likely to have a powerful influence over a long period of time.

THE THERAPEUTIC PROCESS

To begin the therapeutic process, we must learn to recognize and evaluate our own actions and responses in given situations. It is important to know how we feel about ourselves. We must understand ourselves and like ourselves before we can begin to understand and like others.

What Is Self-Awareness?

Self-awareness is being aware of oneself as an individual. It includes all the beliefs a person has with respect to behavior. It is the mental image of the self, and may be realistic or unrealistic. It is also changeable and is affected by each of the influences previously mentioned. Self-awareness begins to form at a very early age and is well established by the age of 6.

Before going further, take time now to complete the "I am" statements in Exercise 1 in this chapter. This exercise will stimulate your thinking about yourself and assist you in making some assessments about yourself as well. Do you accept yourself as you are now, or would you like to make some changes?

While we cannot do much to change many of the things that influences our lives, we *can* recognize their presence, evaluate their effect, and begin to initiate change as necessary. One way to do this is through self-assessment.

The Value of Self-Assessment

The value of *self-assessment* is that it helps us determine who we are, as seen by self and by others. It is a tool to illustrate both positive and negative characteristics so that changes may be implemented. These changes encourage growth and keep us from becoming stagnant. Self-assessment gives us the power to accept or alter these changes.

Each of us has three selves living within one body: the *ideal self*, the *public self*, and the *real self*. The *ideal self* is the person we think we should be and the person we would like to become. The *public self* is how we want others to see us. We may have many public selves, depending upon the circle of people with whom we have contact. The public self is our reputation. The *real self* is the inner, natural self, authentic and spontaneous. When you are most true to yourself and transparent to others, you are being your real self.

In order to have positive self-acceptance, there must be a congruency between all three selves. All three must be balanced and there must be a good feeling about each dimension.

Complete Exercise 2, which is related to the three selves, to assist you in determining how you personally feel about the three dimensions of your self. What did you learn about yourself? Can you make any changes in your life to facilitate growth?

PROFESSIONAL APPLICATION

After reflecting on yourself and how you relate to others, an important concept must be considered. Are you the type of person most suited for a career in a health care profession? Some members of helping professions give so much of themselves to their clients and their work that they quickly become disillusioned and suffer burnout. Others remain so aloof and detached from their work and their clients' needs that they can become rude and disinterested. Neither situation is appropriate, or successful.

Health care professionals should ask themselves the following simple questions:

1. *Do you genuinely enjoy helping people in a therapeutic manner?* This implies that you have the technical skills and knowledge to help people solve their problems, and that you do so without the need to create more power for yourself.

2. *Can you feel comfortable assuming a "servant" role for those in need?* "Servant" does not imply "slave," but you must genuinely enjoy serving the needs of others.

3. *Will you be able to treat any person as a "guest" no matter what their special circumstances may be?* Remember, your employment is dependent upon a satisfied customer.

4. *Can you be open to people and accept their differences?* Even though your personal lifestyle might be quite the opposite, can you be accepting and unflappable? Are you tolerant? Can you keep your opinions to yourself?

5. *Can you be firm, yet gentle?* Procedures you perform may cause discomfort and/or pain, but your verbal and nonverbal communication must convey both firmness and gentleness.

6. *Can you keep yourself out of a codependent relationship with those you help?* People in helping professions may adopt a hostile attitude toward their clients after so many years of rescuing and giving so much. Many health care professionals are harried and overcommitted, and so locked into a caretaker role that they feel dismayed and rejected when they cannot "save" someone.

Prior to considering the numerous aspects of communications more closely, read the following scenario, and ask yourself how you might respond as a health care professional. What does your response reveal about you?

❧ CASE STUDY ❧

When a young woman discovers she is pregnant, the news can be either joyous or devastating. For one young woman named Elaine, it was not good news. She was unemployed, had no money, and was very much alone. Her desperation took her to the welfare office. Elaine realized she needed proper care for herself and the baby.

As time passed, she realized that she did not have what she wanted for her baby—a place to live, two loving parents, proper medical attention, and a mother who was emotionally mature and financially secure. Elaine chose adoption as the best solution. She finally selected an adoption agency after investigating several.

After several weeks and no opportunity to identify for the agency the kind of parents she would like for her baby, and little or no prenatal care assistance, she left the agency and decided to work through a private attorney for the adoption.

After only two conversations with the attorney, who explained his services for birth mothers and adoptive parents, her self-esteem improved. She completed a detailed questionnaire describing herself and her family. She completed an equally detailed summary of the kind of qualities she was looking for in parents for her baby. The attorney insisted she receive prenatal care and provided her with the proper resources. Soon he matched her with a set of prospective parents.

Even though the decision had been made prior to the baby's birth about who the adoptive parents would be, Elaine knew the final separation would be very difficult. Elaine's obstetrician and his office staff knew of her

continues

Case Study continued

decision. They described for her the procedure at the hospital, and even arranged for her not to be in the maternity wing. But at no time did they discourage her from seeing her baby or deny her the rights of any other expectant mother.

At the time of the baby's delivery, the reckoning came. The comments and the nonverbal actions of the hospital staff would make the difference. She was given the same treatment any other expectant mother would receive, and her best friend and birthing coach were ushered into the delivery room with her. When the baby was born, the delivery room nurse asked Elaine if she wanted to hold the baby. When Elaine said no, the nurse held Elaine's hand, smiled, and told her that was fine. She could see the baby, hold the baby, even feed the baby at any time, if she wanted.

Later that day, Elaine would appear at the nursery room window, asking to see her baby. During the next 24 hours, while the attorney and adoptive parents were being notified, Elaine would hold, feed, and change this baby girl she was about to release. The adoptive parents had flown over 1,500 miles to receive the baby, so they were still a few hours away when it was time for Elaine to be discharged from the hospital.

Elaine and the adoptive parents had agreed that the baby should not go to a foster home for even a few moments, so the nurses made arrangements for Elaine to remain in the hospital, without additional charge, until the adoptive parents arrived.

The tearful exchange took place later, and Elaine gave over her daughter to be loved and cared for by the adoptive parents. One nurse assisted the ecstatic adoptive mother, while another walked the birth mother through the hospital dismissal. Elaine was deeply saddened by her loss, but she was not broken or ashamed.

This story is repeated every day around the country. How different might it be if the comments and actions of the health care professional were critical and judgmental? Can you cite examples of both social and therapeutic communications? A closer look at how communication takes place will help assess therapeutic communications.

THE COMMUNICATION CYCLE

Communication is the sending and receiving of messages. Sometimes we are aware or conscious of the messages being sent or received and sometimes we are not. We are, however, always sending and receiving them.

Communication is a complex action in which two or more people participate. As shown in Figure 1-1, there are four basic elements involved in the communication cycle: 1) a sender, 2) a message and the channel or mode of communication, 3) a receiver, and 4) feedback.

The Sender

The sender begins the communication cycle by creating or encoding the message. The sender must formulate a clear thought to send. There is great value in choosing words carefully in order to send a clear message to the receiver.

The Message

The message is the content to be communicated. The four channels or modes of communication most pertinent in our everyday exchanges include 1) speaking, 2) listening, 3) gestures or body language, and 4) writing. These may also be categorized into verbal and nonverbal communication.

How we send and how we perceive messages, to a large extent, is based on the influences discussed earlier. Regardless of these influences, the message sent must be adapted to fit the situation and the receiver.

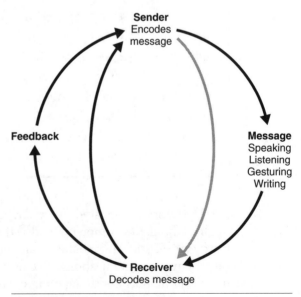

FIGURE 1-1   The communication cycle and channels of communication.

Each of these channels of communication has its appropriateness. In some instances, a written message may be the most effective means of communication; in other cases, spoken communication may be best.

The Receiver

A receiver is the recipient of the sender's message. The receiver must decode the message by evaluating the communication. The primary sensory skill used in verbal communication is listening. The spoken words, as well as the tone and pitch of voice, carry meaning. Any emphasis made by the sender must be fully understood by the receiver for the message to have meaning.

Feedback

Feedback occurs when the receiver and sender both verify their perception of the message. Feedback may be either verbal or nonverbal. It reveals to the sender whether the message was interpreted accurately, and enhances understanding by verifying and/or clarifying any misunderstanding. Feedback should be succinct, timely, and relevant to the situation.

VERBAL COMMUNICATION

When a message is spoken, there is verbal communication. Mere spoken words, however, carry no message unless the words have meaning. If you overhear a conversation in a language foreign to you, you are a witness to verbal communication, but you may not understand the message.

The spoken word, to have any meaning, must be understood by all parties to the communication. The book *Legal Nurse Consulting Principles and Practice*, edited by Patricia W. Iyer, identifies the five Cs of communication. They are 1) complete, 2) clear, 3) concise, 4) cohesive, and 5) courteous. These five Cs apply equally well to therapeutic communications.

The message must be *complete*, with all the necessary information given. It appears that the adoption agency first told Elaine she would be able to choose her baby's parents. What she discovered much later in the process was that she would not be able to do so until she had signed papers releasing the baby. The message was incomplete, even misleading, in its detail.

The information given in the message must also be *clear*. It must be spoken in terms understandable to both parties. It is best to enunciate carefully, with good diction, and to keep objects out of and away from your mouth. Verbal communication will be most clear when there is eye contact.

A *concise* message is one that does not include unnecessary information. Imagine how different the message would have been had the delivery room nurse said to Elaine, "Well, you really should hold this baby. She is yours. I'd certainly hold her if she were mine."

A *cohesive* message is logical and in order. It does not jump abruptly from one subject to another. You would not say to a client, "Please remove all your clothes. No, we better weigh you first. Or do you want to give us a urine sample now?" You have confused the receiver and lost his/her attention.

A message must always be *courteous* if it is to be therapeutic. Any time communication is not considerate, there is a risk that the message will be unclear, even not received, because of the defenses likely to be present in either the sender or the receiver.

NONVERBAL COMMUNICATION

Taber's Cyclopedic Dictionary defines body language as the unconscious use of postures, gestures, or other forms of nonverbal expression in communication. **Kinesics** is defined as the systematic study of the body and the use of its static and dynamic position as a means of communication. Nonverbal communication does not involve speaking in words, but uses gestures and mannerisms. Nonverbal communication is the language we learn first. It is learned seemingly automatically, as infants learn to smile in response to a smile or loving touches on the cheek long before they respond verbally. Much of our body language is a learned behavior and is greatly influenced by the culture in which we are raised.

Feelings are communicated quite well nonverbally. Since nonverbal communication is much less subject to conscious control, emotional dimensions are often expressed nonverbally. The body naturally expresses our true, repressed feelings. Most of the negative messages we express nonverbally are unintended. But whether they are intentional or not, the message is relayed. Experts tell us that 70 percent of communication is nonverbal. The tone of voice communicates 23 percent of the message, and only 7 percent of the message is actually communicated in what is said.

Two Key Points to Successful Communication

There are two key points to remember in successful communication.

- First, there must be congruency between the verbal and the nonverbal message. This means the two messages must be in agreement or be consistent with one another. If I verbally tell you I am not angry, but speak in angry tones, have my fists clenched and my face contorted, I am sending a mixed message. Chances are you will believe my nonverbal message rather than the verbal.

- Second, remember that nonverbal cues appear in groups. The grouping of gestures, facial expressions, and postures into nonverbal statements is known as **clustering**. In the previous example, the tone of voice, the gesture of clenched fists, and the facial expression form a nonverbal statement or cluster of cues to true feelings and emotions.

TYPES OF NONVERBAL COMMUNICATION

Facial Expression

Perhaps the most important nonverbal communicator is facial expression. It has been said that the eyes mirror the soul. The eyes can communicate several kinds of messages. Have you ever seen laughter and joy in another's eyes? Have you seen grief or pain reflected in someone's eyes?

Eye contact is another form of facial expression, and is often viewed as a sign of interest in the individual. It provides cues to indicate that what others say is important. A long stare may be interpreted as an invasion of privacy, which creates an uncomfortable, uneasy feeling. A lack of eye contact in Western culture is usually interpreted to mean a lack of involvement, or avoidance.

Certain movements of the eyebrow seem to indicate questioning, while others may disclose feelings of amusement, surprise, puzzlement, or worry. The manner in which the forehead is wrinkled also sends similar messages.

Touch

Touch is one of the most sensitive means of communication. Touch is often used to express deep feelings that are impossible to express verbally, and can be a very powerful means of communication.

For all health care professionals, many tasks involve touching the client. Most clients will understand and accept the touching behavior, as it is related to the medical setting. Some clients, however, are not comfortable being touched, so sensitivity is essential. It is helpful to tell clients when, where, and how they are to be touched during an examination. Explaining all assessments and treatments tends to put individuals at ease. This technique is essential when a client is autistic. An individual with autism has heightened sensory abilities and may attempt to escape sensory overload or a sudden invasion of their personal space. They tend to want to get away from strange people, voices, and equipment. If you find yourself in a helping situation or profession and feel uncomfortable touching, self-assessment or self-awareness may be necessary.

Touch is often synonymous with reassurance, understanding, and caring. It is important to assess our level of comfort, and that of the client, in relation to the use of touch. When we are comfortable using touch and when we are sensitive to a client's level of acceptance to touch, touch can be used in a therapeutic manner.

Personal Space

Personal space is the distance at which individuals are comfortable with others. It may be determined by sociocultural influences. Personal space can be thought of as the invisible fence no one can see. However, the *way* in which we define boundaries *is* evident to others.

We feel threatened when others invade our personal space without our consent. Many individuals have well-defined personal space boundaries. Examples of personal space in Western culture are listed for your consideration.

Intimate	—	touching to 1½ feet
Personal	—	1½ to 4 feet
Social	—	4 to 12 feet (most often observed)
Public	—	12 to 15 feet

Many cultures uphold these four categories of spatial relationships; however, the distances may vary from one culture to another.

Many medically related tasks involve invading another's personal space. It is beneficial to explain procedures that intrude on another's space before beginning the procedure. This gives the client some control, and a sense of dignity and worth.

Position

When speaking with a client, it is helpful to maintain a close but comfortable position. Standing over a client denotes superiority, while too much distance may be interpreted as being exclusive or avoiding. Movement toward a client usually indicates warmth, liking, interest, acceptance, and trust. Moving away may suggest dislike, disinterest, boredom, indifference, suspicion, or impatience (see Figure 1-2).

Posture

Like distance, posture is important to the health care professional. Individuals in threatening situations usually tense, but tend to relax in a non-threatening environment. Posture can be used as a barometer for feelings. For example, sitting with the limbs crossed over one's chest sends a message of closure and avoidance; leaning back in a chair with the arms up and hands clasped behind the head indicates an openness to suggestions.

Slumped shoulders may signal depression, discouragement, or in some cases even pain. It is important to validate the messages before

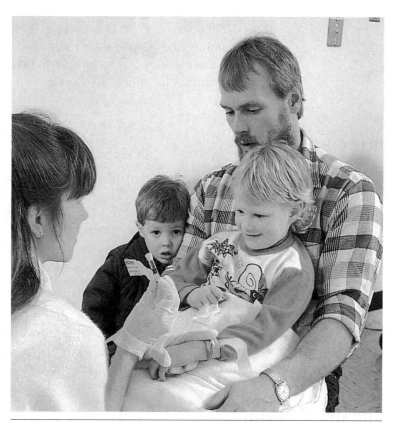

FIGURE 1-2 Positive posture and position encourage therapeutic communication. (Courtesy of Carl Howard/Albany Medical Center)

continuing a procedure. For example, you may ask the client, "Are you comfortable?" or "Is this position too painful?" Technicians must be careful to be in tune to the client's physical comfort.

Gestures/Mannerisms

Most everyone uses gestures or "talks" with their hands to some degree. Gestures are useful in emphasizing ideas, in creating and holding others' attention, and in relieving stress. Some common gestures and their meanings might be these:

Finger-tapping	—	impatience, nervousness
Shrugged shoulders	—	indifference, discouragement
Rubbing the nose	—	puzzlement
Whitened knuckles and clenched fists	—	anger
Fidgeting	—	nervousness

It is important to recognize that nonverbal communication helps understanding, and frequently is more powerful than verbal communication. It is also more enduring and has more persuasive power than verbal communication. The nonverbal message is more quickly believed than the verbal message.

WORD OF CAUTION

It must be remembered, however, that nonverbal communication can easily be misinterpreted. The folded arms may mean the person is cold, not closed to communication. The wrinkled brow may indicate the person has a headache, not a questioning or doubting attitude. Look for congruency between verbal and nonverbal communication for a clear message. Do not make assumptions.

In the earlier scenario, when the delivery room nurse asked Elaine if she would like to hold the baby, the verbal and nonverbal messages were congruent. When Elaine said no, the nurse held Elaine's hand, smiled, and told her that was fine. Together, the cluster of mannerisms used by the delivery room nurse said, "I understand, I care, and your response is appropriate."

LISTENING SKILLS

Listening is often identified as the passive aspect of communication. However, if done well, listening is very active. Good listeners have their eyes upon the speaker, are attentive, and are aware of the nonverbal messages as well as the verbal information coming from the sender. Effective listening requires concentration.

Therapeutic listening includes listening with a "third ear": that is, being aware of what the client is *not* saying or picking up on hints as to the real message. In the scenario of Mrs. Nelson at the beginning of this section, her primary-care physician was either unaware of the nonverbal cues and hints being made or chose to see them as unimportant.

The health care professional should have three listening goals: 1) to improve listening skills sufficiently so that clients are heard accurately; 2) to listen for what is not being said or for information transmitted only by hints; and 3) to determine how accurately the message has been received.

A technique used by many and suggested by professionals is the ability to paraphrase the client's message or statement. This technique allows the receiver of the message to return the message to the sender, perhaps worded differently, allowing the sender to acknowledge the accuracy of the message.

Sender: "Will I be able to use my medical coupons for prenatal care in your clinic?"

Receiver: "You're concerned about whether our doctor accepts medical coupons for payment."

Sender: "That's correct. I have no money. My baby will be adopted, but I know we both need proper medical care."

Receiver: "Our office does take medical coupons, and you will receive the best of care. Would you like to make an appointment?"

This example shows both active listening and therapeutic communication skills. The office assistant heard both concerns—the monetary concern and the concern for proper care.

Health care professionals must be prudent in how they use active listening techniques, however. It is not appropriate to paraphrase everything the client says; otherwise the client begins to feel stupid, or believes the professional has a hearing problem.

One of the greatest barriers to listening occurs when receivers find themselves thinking about something else while trying to listen. It is difficult to try to concentrate on what is being said when the mind is wandering. When this happens, pull concentration back to the sender, apologize if necessary, and continue with the communication.

There is a time in communication, in listening, when silence is appropriate. So many times health care professionals try to "fix" everything with a recommendation, a prescription, or even advice. Sometimes none of those things are necessary. The client simply needs someone to listen, to acknowledge the difficulty, and to remember that the client is not helpless in finding a solution to the problem.

Skill in communication takes years of practice and frequent review. It will never become perfect; the goal is to become *better* at it with each passing day. Communication is and always will be the very basis for any therapeutic relationship.

INFLUENCE OF TECHNOLOGY ON COMMUNICATION

There will always be face-to-face communication, telephone conversations between two individuals, and paper communication in the health care setting, but electronic mail (e-mail), facsimile (fax) messaging, video and teleconferences, and conference calls among three or more individuals are increasingly common in health care. Cellular telephones, personal digital assistants (PDAs), and laptop computers can be linked to a network for Internet access or communication with satellite facilities from almost anywhere in the world. In this environment, however, the content of the message is likely to be examined for credibility without any of the nonverbal cues such as eye contact, facial expression, or posture. Communication interactions required when using this technology require special training.

The use of *electronic mail (e-mail)* is popular in the health care setting, both in communication with clients and in communication with colleagues. E-mail sends, receives, stores, and forwards messages over computer networks. At the convenience of the sender, e-mail communication is sent to one person or a number of individuals at one time. It is also read at the convenience of the receiver. Clients are particularly interested in the use of electronic mail (sometimes called clinical e-mail) for such things as prescription refill, appointment scheduling, information updates, or simple requests that normally would not require a visit and are more convenient than placing a telephone call, leaving a message, and waiting for a response.

E-mail communication is used only for active clients who generally have been examined within the last six months. No information can be provided through electronic mail without the clients' release of information to do so. Only clients can determine what, if any, personal health information (PHI) can be shared. The **Health Insurance Portability and Accountability Act (HIPAA)** is very specific in its guidelines for electronic transmission of client information. It is not the purpose of this text to detail HIPAA guidelines, but the Web site for the Department of Health and Human Services is helpful (www.hhs.gov/o cr/hipaa/). General guidelines for all e-mail etiquette include the following:

- Be concise and to the point.

- Respond in a timely fashion and answer all questions.

- Use proper spelling and grammar.

- Do not attach unnecessary files.

- Do not write in CAPITALS.

- Add disclaimers to the e-mail.

- Read any e-mail prior to sending.

- Any clinical e-mail regarding a client should be copied and placed in the chart.

Fax messaging uses telephone lines to transmit data from one fax machine to another. It is often used for referrals, insurance approvals, and informal correspondence. The same standards of confidentiality for any client information identified in an e-mail exist for fax communication. Fax machines are likely to be placed in a centralized area where unauthorized individuals may see documents being sent by fax. A cover sheet should be included that stipulates the information is for the intended recipient only. Fax messaging saves the time and effort of copying and mailing a document, allowing the sender to keep the original while providing the recipient with an exact duplicate.

Satellite *video* and *teleconferencing* are used to share information, receive education and training in a particular field of health care, or conduct a meeting to make certain decisions. A video conference will allow participants to see one another and interact almost as if the individuals were together in one room. A teleconference consists of a group of individuals connected by only the telephone. Both video and teleconferences can become difficult to manage if more than 10 participants are included. A telephone conference should be limited to 30 minutes or less, since it is difficult for participants to concentrate while looking into space for any longer period of time.

Effective video and teleconferencing, as well as telephone conference calls, include some basic rules of conduct:

- One person is the facilitator and is responsible for keeping the meeting on track.

- Come prepared with necessary documents or information that is to be shared.

- Before speaking, remember that everyone may not recognize your voice or know who you are; always begin with "This is _____."

- Silence is not bad. Facial expressions may not be evident, and someone may be formulating a question prior to speaking. Also, do not assume silence means consent.

- Stay focused on the meeting. The conscious mind cannot perform some other task and give full attention to the meeting at the same time.

TEAM COMMUNICATION

The use of technological communication is key to effective team interaction. Health care professionals in any major health care system should receive specialized training in the facility's protocol for the use and dissemination of all communications. Even in much smaller health care facilities, care must be given to communication among its employees.

There must be guidelines or policies on what can be communicated via e-mail, fax, video, and teleconference. Some simple rules to consider follow:

- Do not use e-mail if a walk into an adjacent office for a face-to-face communication is possible.

- Reserve two to four times daily to check e-mail; notify others of your decision. Otherwise, you can become a "slave" to the technology.

- Answer e-mails within a 24-hour time period or less; create a response message when you are out of the facility for any period of time.

- Remember that e-mail is not private.

- Be careful what you forward and seek permission to do so.

- Do not use the facility's computer for personal e-mail.

- Use "flags" and "Important" sparingly.

- Do not send libelous, defamatory, offensive, racist, or obscene remarks.

In order to communicate effectively as a team member, take time to develop skills that will ensure levels of trust, and to build into the team a sense of worth and importance. Consideration also must be given to cultural diversity and to understanding ways in which other cultures communicate. For example, during a business meeting, Americans prefer to be seated either face-to-face or at right angles to each other. Asian cultures prefer side-by-side positions. Americans generally follow Maslow's Hierarchy of Needs (refer to Appendix A), with self-actualization as the pinnacle, whereas Asian society emphasizes belonging.

SUMMARY

Understanding self and the basic components of communication is vital to establishing a therapeutic relationship with clients, who likely come to the "helping relationship" with a number of barriers that impede communication. Clients may be anxious, experiencing pain, or acutely ill. Communication that understands these barriers, keeps in mind the communication cycle, and comes from health care professionals who know and understand themselves will help empower clients to be full participants in the client-professional relationship. Remember, too, that effective communication skills require special attention when interacting with others using electronic e-mail or sending fax documents.

EXERCISES

Exercise 1

Read the following statements and select the 10 statements you think best describe you. Then select 8 statements you think *least* describe you. Ask a friend to indicate the statements they think describe you the best, and the least.

"I AM" STATEMENTS

I am a perfectionist.

I am dependable.

I am reserved.

I am realistic.

I am a happy person.

I am well-liked.

I am easily hurt.

I am impulsive.

I am self-conscious.

I am secure.

I am sympathetic.

I am able to express emotions.

I am unpredictable.

I am often opinionated.

I am creative.

I am self-reliant.

I am naive.

I am sometimes incompetent.

I am self-sacrificing.

I am generous.

I am able to live by rules.

I am a worrier.

I am shy.

I am intelligent.

I have a good self-image.

I am afraid of failure.

I am hard to get along with.

I am competitive.

I am ambitious.

I am courageous.

I am an understanding person.

I am often depressed.

I am easygoing.

I am socially adept.

I am often lonely.

I am in control.

I am socially inept.

I am disorganized.

I am a well-groomed person.

I am an attractive person.

I am selfish.

I am a decision maker.

I am not very attractive.

I am usually confident.

I am precise.

I am realistic.

I am overprotective.

I am energetic.

I am tolerant.

I am responsible for myself.

I am a people person.

I am assertive.

I am fickle.

I am argumentative.

I am fun-loving.

I am often suspicious of others.

I am demanding of myself.

I often feel insecure.

I am generally trusting.

I can usually make a decision.

I am oversensitive.

I am poised.

Exercise 2

Using the columns provided, list adjectives that describe how you perceive your three selves.

Ideal Self	Public Self	Real Self
Ask the question, "What kind of person do I wish to become?"	You may wish to ask someone who knows you to describe you.	What do you really feel inside?

Exercise 3

Write a paragraph discussing a recent incident, preferably personal, in which a communicator failed to communicate what was intended. Analyze why this happened and how it could have been avoided.

REVIEW QUESTIONS

Multiple Choice

1. Human relations skills
   - **a.** require specific and technical training.
   - **c.** are interpersonal skills seen in professional and personal relationships.
   - **b.** are all that is necessary in the health care setting.
   - **d.** are not exhibited through nonverbal communication.

2. Therapeutic communication
   - **a.** requires specific, well-defined professional skills.
   - **c.** takes place only in verbal communication.
   - **b.** is not influenced by personal feelings of self.
   - **d.** does not change with culture.

3. Each individual has three selves; they are
   - **a.** social self, real self, and hidden self.
   - **c.** social self, ideal self, and real self.
   - **b.** ideal self, hidden self, and public self.
   - **d.** ideal self, public self, and real self.

4. The fourth basic element in the communication cycle
   - **a.** verifies the message.
   - **c.** is the recipient of the sender's message.
   - **b.** may be verbal or nonverbal.
   - **d.** both a and b above.

5. The five Cs of communication are
   - **a.** complete, clear, concise, courteous, congruent.
   - **c.** correct, concise, concrete, complete, courteous.
   - **b.** complete, clear, concise, cohesive, courteous.
   - **d.** correct, clear, complete, courteous, congruent.

6. Experts tell us that _____% of communication is nonverbal.
   - **a.** 32%
   - **c.** 70%
   - **b.** 7%
   - **d.** 93%

7. Effective listening
   - a. is the passive part of communication.
   - b. requires concentration.
   - c. comes naturally to most individuals.
   - d. pays attention only to the spoken word.

8. Communication using modern technological advances does not easily evaluate
   - a. cultural diversity.
   - b. nonverbal cues.
   - c. listening skills.
   - d. content credibility.

FOR FURTHER CONSIDERATION

1. On a sheet of paper, identify and describe yourself as briefly and as fully as possible. (For instance: I am a woman, a mother, a grandmother; I am Native American; I am a sister to four siblings, etc.) For each descriptive, explain how to relate to an individual who is just the opposite, or quite different. (For instance, a man, a father, a grandfather, or someone who is not a parent; a man from East India, etc.) How do you communicate professionally and therapeutically, realizing these differences?

2. Go to the section in this chapter on Professional Application on p. 9 and respond to question 3. Identify how you might be able to treat someone as a "guest" in a health care setting when he or she is someone you would not have as a guest in your home. List the reasons why this individual would *not* be a guest in your home. What do you do to remain therapeutic? Do you have any prejudices to reconsider?

3. Can you be sympathetic with Elaine in the second scenario? Could you give up a child for adoption? If not, and you are the health care professional assigned to Elaine during delivery, what will you do to communicate therapeutically?

CASE STUDIES

Case Study 1

Zena is a home health care aide. She is assisting an 83-year-old woman to dress herself when the woman stumbles and slumps to the floor. As Zena gets down to help her, the woman begins to cry, and says, "I am so useless; I can't do anything anymore." What should Zena do? What might Zena say?

Case Study 2

You are a receptionist in a skilled nursing facility. You are expecting a new resident this afternoon. He is an 85-year-old gentleman who is coming for several days of rehabilitation prior to release to his home. His wife, aged 82, is awaiting hip replacement surgery and walks with a cane. You happen to look out the glass door to see a taxi pull up. You see that this is your new admit and his wife. The taxi driver does not get out of the car or open the door for his passengers. What are the passengers feeling at this point? What will you do? What kind of skills will you demonstrate?

RESOURCES

Antai-Otong, D. (2003). *Psychiatric nursing: biological and behavioral concepts*. Clifton Park, NY: Thomson Delmar Learning.

Desmond, J., & Copeland, L. R. (2000). *Communicating with today's patient*. San Francisco, CA: Jossey-Bass.

Lindh, W. Q., Pooler, M., Tamparo, C. D., & Dahl, B. (2006). *Administrative medical assisting* (3rd ed.). Clifton Park, NY: Thomson Delmar Learning.

Patricia W. I. (Ed.). (2002). *Legal nurse consulting principles and practice*. Boca Raton, FL: CRC Press.

Schuster, P. M. (2000). *Communication*. Philadelphia, PA: F. A. Davis Company.

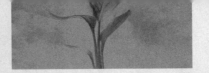

CHAPTER

2

Multicultural Therapeutic Communication

CHAPTER OBJECTIVES

The learner should strive to meet the following chapter objectives and demonstrate an understanding of the facts and principles presented in this chapter through written and oral communication.

- Define key terms as presented in the glossary.

- Identify and explain three important factors that help build multicultural communication.

- List and describe a minimum of five techniques to employ when communicating with individuals of other cultures.

- Discuss barriers to multicultural therapeutic communication and suggest ways these barriers may be decreased or eliminated.

- Identify at least three steps that may be taken to learn more about other cultures.

- Identify cultural biases and prejudices that may be experienced in today's health care facilities.

- Differentiate between low- and high-context communication styles.

- Describe differences in the caregiving structure of various cultures.

- Discuss the impact of time focus—future, present, or past—on various cultures.

- Describe Maslow's Hierarchy of Needs and its relationship to time focus.

- Compare and contrast the cultural and religious backgrounds of various cultures.
- Discuss the differences in religion-based cultures.
- Discuss recognized types of medicine: Western medicine, holistic medicine, Oriental medicine, and folk medicine.
- Discuss cultural brokering and its benefits to health care.
- Discuss guidelines to follow when working with a medical interpreter.

OPENING CASE STUDY

Beatrice completed her medical assistant training near her hometown in rural Wisconsin and, because of better opportunities for employment, moved to Newark, New Jersey to be able to follow her career goal of becoming a physician assistant. She was hired as an MA in a clinic in a predominantly middle-class, working neighborhood populated primarily by Puerto Ricans and African-Americans. While Beatrice was preparing a client for examination that she thought her previous doctor was very "bad". Beatrice was shocked and did not know what to say or do about this statement.

INTRODUCTION

The opening case study illustrates a communication problem directly related to cultural differences between the client and the medical assistant. The material in this chapter generalizes cultural differences that may be encountered in the United States, and provides a beginning knowledge base for understanding cultures outside the mainstream.

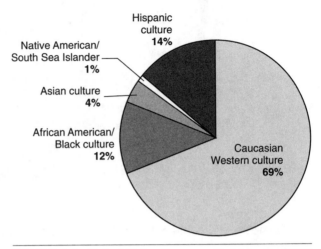

FIGURE 2-1   United States Demographic Make-Up (2000 Census).

Successfully achieving multicultural therapeutic communication requires consideration of the cultural background of the client. Approximately one-third of the population of the United States come from a culture other than mainstream American; i.e. Caucasian, English-speaking, Judeo-Christian. See Figure 2-1. Some of the predominant ethnic/religious cultural characteristics that may affect therapeutic communication are discussed in this chapter. Entire books could be written on this subject. In this text, the authors generalize similar cultures together to establish a knowledge base to be used in understanding clients of ethnic diversity. Medical professionals working within a specific cultural community should seek further information relating to that particular culture or individual client. In many instances, health care professionals can develop rapport with their ethnically diverse clients by simply demonstrating an interest in their culture and background.

DEVELOPING MULTICULTURAL COMMUNICATION

Culture is a pattern of many concepts, beliefs, values, habits, skills, instruments, and art of a given group of people in a given period. Multicultural communication is the ability to communicate effectively with individuals of other cultures while recognizing one's own personal cultural biases and prejudices and putting them aside. Three important actions to promote multicultural communication are 1) to become knowledgeable about the beliefs and values of different cultures, 2) to develop techniques that build and foster multicultural communication, and 3) to recognize barriers to multicultural communication.

Therapeutic communication takes place between a person who has a specific need, no matter what their culture, and a person who is skilled in techniques that can identify, resolve, or satisfy that need. Therapeutic communication is goal-oriented. When health care professionals engage in multicultural therapeutic communication, clients from different cultures are assisted with their health-related goals and their personal and cultural values are respected.

BARRIERS TO MULTICULTURAL THERAPEUTIC COMMUNICATION

Joan Luckmann, in her book entitled *Transcultural Communication in Health Care*, identifies eight barriers to therapeutic transcultural communication: 1) lack of knowledge; 2) fear and distrust; 3) racism; 4) prejudice, bias and ethnocentrism; 5) stereotyping; 6) health care rituals; 7) language; and 8) differences in perceptions and expectations. The following paragraphs explore each of these barriers and discuss tactics for overcoming or diminishing them within health care settings.

Lack of Knowledge

In order to provide culturally sensitive health care, health care professionals must understand and take into consideration the cultural differences of their clients. The first step is to learn more about clients' cultures. Begin by making a list of the cultures served and conduct a systematic study of each. Libraries contain autobiographies, biographies, novels, and essays related to various cultures. The Internet is another useful resource. Television provides travel documentary programs that are both interesting and informative. Enjoy a restaurant meal with a different cultural cuisine. Consider involving staff in a culture-of-the-month study. At the end of the month, an in-house luncheon could be shared, with each staff member bringing a food contribution representing that culture. Sharing the knowledge learned broadens the base for each staff member and builds a comfort level for interacting with clients of that culture.

Fear and Distrust

When meeting someone from another culture, one's first response or reaction may be reservation, because the other person looks, dresses, or seems different, or may communicate in a different language or dialect. Such a reserved attitude can become fear or concern because of a lack of understanding of the culture. Confusion from the messages being sent, verbally or nonverbally, may lead to feelings of dislike and distrust.

Knowing more about the other culture helps to dispel these emotions. When the cause of this fear and distrust is recognized, cross-cultural communication becomes easier.

Racism

Race includes any of the major biological divisions of mankind, distinguished by color and texture of hair, color of skin and eyes, stature, bodily proportions, etc. **Racism** implies racial discrimination, segregation, persecution, and domination. Individuals, cultural groups, or institutions can experience racism. Racism is present in American health care, based on studies conducted at Johns Hopkins University in 2000. Most everyone has some racial biases toward one or more cultures or races. This is not unusual, as it has only been about three decades since racism in the United States became politically incorrect. Actual racism or perceived racism results in fear and distrust between client and health care provider, with a resulting negative impact on therapeutic communication. It is beyond the scope of this text to resolve the problem, but it is possible to highlight what individuals can do to become more racially tolerant.

The elimination of racism in an individual begins with knowledge and the examination of conscious and unconscious attitudes regarding race and culture. The next step is a commitment to changing the attitude(s). Engaging in open and honest discussions with others helps in recognizing personal feelings on the subject and reinforces a commitment to eliminate racism.

Bias, Prejudice, and Ethnocentrism

Bias is a slant toward a particular belief. **Prejudice** is an opinion or judgment that is formed before all of the facts are known; prejudice is usually preconceived and unfavorable. Body language may unconsciously transmit bias or prejudice. **Ethnocentrism** is the belief that one's own culture and traditions are better than those of another. Health care professionals must be willing to acknowledge their personal biases, prejudices, and ethnocentrism as blocks to therapeutic communication. They must be willing to accept the uniqueness of each individual's culture.

Common biases and prejudices in today's society include

- A preference for Western medicine
- Physicians chosen according to gender
- Prejudice related to a person's sexual preference
- Discrimination based on race or religion

- Hostile attitudes toward individuals with different value systems
- A belief that people who cannot afford health care should receive less care than someone who can pay for full services.

Stereotyping

Stereotyping consists of attributing an unvarying description or pattern to a person with no allowance for individuality. Stereotyping says that all individuals of a particular culture are exactly alike. This philosophy is not true, even though individuals may share many cultural characteristics. It is important to recognize how personal perceptions may distort interactions with other cultures. Saying such things as "Mexicans always," or "black people never," or any comments that stereotype a group of people can be very serious, and indicates a need for self-examination.

Health Care Rituals

Health care **rituals** are standardized procedures or protocols followed during a client visit. Some rituals are necessary from a medical point of view and others are not. For example, when children visit a dentist, parents may be asked to wait in the reception area during the examination. While this may be protocol, it may not be well received by individuals or clients from cultures who expect and feel more comfortable with the entire family coming along. Health care professionals must consider the rationale for such procedures and make exceptions when appropriate. The child coming for a first-time visit may need the security of the parent or caregiver during the examination. The parent or caregiver will be more comfortable staying behind at the next visit, knowing the child is familiar with what is going to happen and having seen professionals interacting with the child.

Language

Non-English-speaking clients may require the use of an interpreter for effective communication. In selecting an interpreter, the **dialect** of the client must be considered. For example, Chinese dialects may include Mandarin, Cantonese, or Shanghainese. Each dialect is unique, with its own cultural nuances. Dialect, as well as **regionalism**, may also be encountered with English-speaking clients. Clients from Scotland, while speaking English, can have a brogue that is almost incomprehensible to Americans. Another language barrier compounding communication problems is the unique meanings given to different words based on the experience, culture, and ethnicity of the client. African Americans sometimes use a street language called **Ebonics**. The example in the opening case study, referring to the doctor as "bad," is an example of Ebonics, and actually is a complimentary statement meaning "very good."

When communicating with culturally diverse populations, people who speak English as a second language (ESL), also referred to as English speakers of other languages (ESOL), will be encountered. Many ESL clients have not learned to *think* in English and must first translate the English words into their native language, process the thought, and then translate it back into English before responding. This will require the health care professional to speak rather slowly, to use simple terms, and to realize there may be a delay in receiving a response from the client.

It is also important to remember that the process of communicating differs among cultures: It involves *how* the message is said, *when* it is said, and *why* it is said. Understanding various cultures and their values, beliefs, and communication styles will greatly enhance effective multicultural communication.

When working with non-English-speaking clients or clients with limited English-speaking skills, it is vital that these limitations not be perceived as limited intelligence. In their own language, clients may be able to fluently discuss their health care needs. It is only the language limitation that gets in the way of understanding. Also, just because a client does not understand English, there is no reason to speak louder. Use a normal tone of voice and speak a little slower, while enunciating each word clearly and using simpler vocabulary words. Allow clients extra time to process what is said and to form a response.

 STOP AND CONSIDER

Write your thoughts on how you would respond to the opening case study about Beatrice and cultural awareness. After you have studied this entire chapter, review your first thoughts on this question. Are there any changes you would initiate, and why?

Perceptions and Expectations

Perceptions are insights or intuitions of which we are consciously aware. Perception takes sensory data and personalizes it into images of reality. Closely study Figure 2-2. Two entirely different images emerge, depending on whether the eye is focused on the image or the white background. In health care, perceptions must be verified and validated in order to prevent misunderstandings. For example, clients from other cultures may not understand why they should drink cold fluids when they have a cold.

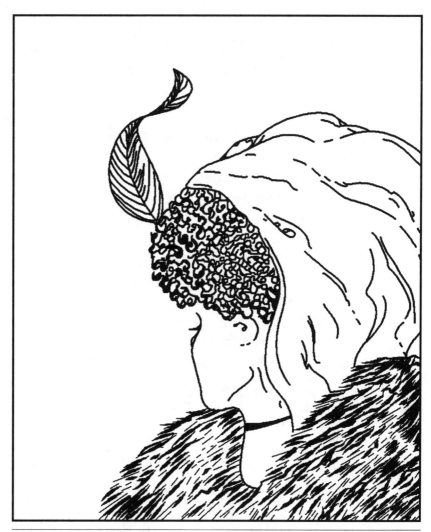

FIGURE 2-2 Young Girl and Old Woman Optical Illusion.

Their holistic practice would be to treat the cold with a hot drink or food. (See Ancient Greek Influence on Culture section on p. 48.)

Expectations are the events we anticipate based on experience or communication. We usually expect clients to use the same communication style and language as we do. In some Asian countries, it is not polite to have eye contact with someone who is older or considered superior, yet in Western culture, it is common to have eye contact. When expectations do not match with reality, confusion and misinterpretation frequently occur and therapeutic communication is stifled.

The Therapeutic Response

When interacting with clients of different cultures, the following basic communication techniques will be helpful.

- Know as much as possible about the culture's communication style.

- Approach the client slowly and respectfully. Do not touch or offer to shake hands with the client until you have assessed their cultural background.

- Create an atmosphere that is comfortable and respects the client's personal space.

- Allow sufficient time, and try not to rush the client.

- Listen to the words clients use to express concerns. Incorporate these words into your verbal responses.

- Recognize and respect the culture's nonverbal mannerisms and gestures.

- Use reflecting questions or statements to validate the feelings and concerns of the client. This encourages clients to share more completely.

- Ask questions of clients to assess fully their cultural background and any clues to cultural barriers in medical treatment. (See Table 2-1)

- Do not jump to conclusions based on your own culture and belief systems.

TABLE 2-1 Cultural Domains and Their Content

A good place to start in defining the cultural characteristics of a client is to utilize some of the cultural domains identified in the Purnell model for cultural competence, and to formulate questions to define each domain. Five of the twelve domains in the Purnell model are appropriate to multicultural therapeutic communication. The following table defines the domains and the points that describe each domain.

Communication	Language spoken
	Context
	Volume or tone of speech
	Body language
	Sensitivity to touch
	Comfort zone
	Eye contact
Family Roles in Health Care	Head of household and gender roles
	Principal caregiver
	Role of extended family
Health Care Practices	Focus of health care
	Traditional practices

(continues)

TABLE 2-1 *(continued)*	
	Folk medicine/holistic medicine
	Magic/religious/traditional beliefs
	Pain
	Self medication/prevention
	Acceptance of medical procedures
	Expectations
Health Care Practitioners	Perception of practitioners
	Gender of practitioners
	Folk practitioners
Spirituality	Spirituality and health
	Use of prayer
	Meaning of life
	Religion/religious practices
	Religious taboos

Each of the domains can be identified by observation, by research, or by asking questions related to each of the elements making up a domain. It might be possible to have the client complete a questionnaire to find out many of the answers. This would also evaluate the client's ability to follow instructions and to communicate in writing.

MANIFESTATIONS OF CULTURAL DIVERSITY

Culture is a major influence on communication between medical personnel and clients. The following sections attempt to identify some of the culturally induced barriers to communication. The text does not completely characterize any given culture, nor is it meant to characterize each individual client. The emphasis is on generalization of groups, to the extent that is possible. This provides a basis for an understanding of various cultures.

Communication Context

Communication context refers to the style of communication used by a speaker. Two styles of communication context are defined: low and high. **Low-context communication** utilizes few environmental or cultural **idioms** to convey an idea or concept, but relies mainly on explicit and highly detailed language. **High-context communication** involves great reliance on body language, reference to objects in the environment, and culturally relevant phraseology to convey an idea. The stereotype of Native American communication shown in old American Westerns exaggerates high-context communication. The preceding sentence is also an example of high-context communication, as it requires cultural knowledge of old American Western movies. High-context communication assumes that the speaker and the listener both have knowledge regarding the subject.

No communication style is superior to another; the important thing to remember is that both the speaker and the listener should be cognizant of the style being used. The high-context style involves painting a word picture based on common experiences shared between the speaker and the listener. If both individuals do not share the same experiences, the word picture is not focused and miscommunication results. Conversely, the low-context style requires that the vocabulary of the listener be at least equal to the spoken vocabulary of the speaker.

People from cultures utilizing different context styles often develop an incorrect impression of each other. Low-context communication is direct and "in your face," while high-context communication is indirect and seems to take forever to reach a conclusion. The high-context speaker is often thought of as being less educated or mentally slow, while the low-context speaker is often thought of as being rude because of the directness of his or her speech. Neither of these perceptions is necessarily correct.

Caregiving Structure

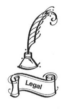

The caregiving structure in a given culture can impact the relationship between medical personnel and clients when it comes to treatment and care. Most adult Caucasians from a Western culture are individualistic and take responsibility for their medical requirements and care. Other cultures, however, do not share this philosophy. This can result in problems with privacy requirements and client adherence to prescribed treatment. In cultures where the principal caregivers are relatives or extended family, the client may find it difficult to understand why these caregivers cannot have access to information about their medical condition and test results without written consent. In some cultures it is quite common for caregivers to accompany a client into the examination room. Special efforts must be taken to ensure compliance with the **Health Insurance Portability and Accountability Act of 1996 (HIPAA)** requirements, while satisfying the client's wishes.

Time Focus

The cultural background, as well as the socioeconomic environment of individuals and cultures, determines their focus regarding time. Time focus can be oriented toward future, present, or past. A review of Maslow's Hierarchy of Needs, found in Appendix A, will be helpful before continuing this section.

Individuals having a *future time focus* are usually confident that their basic needs of food and shelter will be met, and are willing to sacrifice immediate gratification for better returns in the future. Future-oriented individuals are very time conscious and plan out their day and lives in considerable detail. They are usually prompt for appointments and expect the same of others.

Individuals with a *present time focus* are less assured that their needs will be satisfied. It is difficult to develop future plans when the basic items in the Hierarchy of Needs have not been met. It is interesting to note that in cultures where basic needs are provided in abundance, there is also the tendency to have a present time focus. This is possibly due to seeing no reason to improve things in the future. Even after economic status improves, tradition and culture can dictate a present orientation in many groups for generations to come. Artificial limits placed on economic advancement, by a class system or racial or ethnic discrimination, may also cause people to have a present time focus, since improved future status is not an option open to them. Religion can also influence people to adopt a present time focus. Many religions encourage reliance on a spiritual being to provide for daily needs, and believers are encouraged to live day to day. Other religions consider time to be circular, like an endless belt, making time irrelevant. Children in almost all cultures are present focused. Present-oriented people, regardless of the reason for the orientation, do not look on time as being as important as do future-oriented people, and tend to be careless about promptness. It should be clarified that this is not usually out of any disrespect for the other person.

Past time focus is associated with culture and longstanding tradition. Past-oriented people revere traditions and usually honor elders, both living and dead, as well as animals and nature spirits. Asian cultures and Native American cultures frequently exhibit some past orientation. Because past-oriented cultures see time as circular or continuous and repeating, they are not as time conscious as future-oriented people. Because of their respect for elders, however, they usually try to please; hence promptness is a characteristic if they respect the other person or the person is considered educated.

GENERALIZED MANIFESTATIONS
OF CULTURES AND RELIGIONS

Culture and religion have a greater effect on the attitudes relating to medical treatment and therapeutic communication than race and physical characteristics. Culture and religion determine conscious and unconscious beliefs, learned behaviors, and likes and dislikes in clothing and food that develop from life experiences. **Paradigms**, the unconscious part of our culture, result in behavior or choices that may mystify both client and medical personnel. For example, a client's unwillingness to be treated by a female physician may result from the paradigm that all physicians are male. Understanding cultural paradigms may be the greatest challenge encountered during therapeutic communication. In trying to define a culture, individual beliefs and values must not be forgotten. Unless we understand individual aspects of cultures, we will not be able to facilitate effective therapeutic communication. The generalizations portrayed in the following descriptions should not be construed as cultural stereotypes. They are only a starting point in defining a client's culture.

Caucasian, Western Culture

People of Caucasian, Western culture have a high acceptance of **Western medicine**, relying on pharmaceutical products and surgical procedures to treat illness and disease. They lean toward preventive medicine and, generally, are not afraid to question medical opinion. They often take the time to complete extensive research regarding their condition. This enables the client and physician to discuss the problem and various methods of treatment in depth. There is an increasing trend toward integrative medicine, which includes alternative therapies such as natural, holistic, and accommodative medicine. In some rural areas folk or old home cures may be used for all except serious illnesses. This group is characterized by self-reliance, with the client or a member of the immediate family serving as caregiver.

African American, Western Culture

People of African American, Western culture are increasingly similar to people of Caucasian, Western culture. However, there are still many cultural characteristics unique to this group. The greatest difference is in how they focus on time. This group more likely has a present time focus that can result in placing less importance on punctuality, and a lesser disposition toward preventive medicine. The extended family is the predominant caregiver for African Americans; this can present a problem with the HIPAA regulation for privacy unless steps are taken to obtain authorization for release of information from the client. People of African American culture are sometimes distrustful of medical personnel of other cultures. This presents a barrier to successful therapeutic communication when it occurs.

Black, African, or Caribbean Culture

People of Black, African, or Caribbean culture accept Western medicine, but often exhibit a predisposition toward home remedies combined with cures based in spiritualism. The primary caregiver is a relative or a member of the "extended family," which may include people having tribal affiliation. Extended family includes all people the client looks to for trust and support. People of Black, African, or Caribbean culture are basically present time focused and are not likely to place a great amount of importance on punctuality, nor do they lean toward preventive medicine.

Asian Culture

People of Asian culture include many different subcultures (Asian Indian, Chinese, Filipino, Japanese, Korean, Thai, Laotian, and Vietnamese). However, they each have enough similar cultural characteristics to permit treating them as a group. Medical personnel involved in treating primarily one or two of these subcultures may find it beneficial to study their individual cultural characteristics in greater detail. This group, in general, accepts Western medicine; however, it can be strongly influenced by natural or holistic medicine. Confucian principles of mind control over the body, maintaining a balance between natural forces, and eating foods designated "hot or cold" to treat illnesses are often embraced. This culture, along with people in surprising numbers from Western cultures, exhibits strong feeling regarding "saving face" or anything that they perceive makes them feel inferior or ignorant. They will go out of their way to avoid insulting anyone. These characteristics can become a barrier to successful therapeutic communication. People of Asian culture are usually present or past oriented, and display promptness as a symbol of respect. They will frequently smile and agree with a statement by nodding to avoid being disrespectful by challenging or questioning the speaker, or to appear not to understand. People of Asian culture consider mental illness as shameful and deny anything they think suggests a mental condition. While the family is primarily patriarchal, the mother, and sometimes the grandmother, are the primary caregivers. This cultural group is quite private, speaks quietly, and does not believe in touching, especially the head, as it is considered the carrier of the soul and sacred by some.

Native American and South Sea Island Cultures

Native American and South Sea Islanders accept Western medicine. However spirit beliefs, "Mother Nature," or natural control of events in their lives frequently influence them. There is a great reliance on holistic and spiritual cures for illness. They do not frequently speak of illness, as many believe that to do so may cause the problem to occur. This belief is significant to the medical professional, in that it results in an unwillingness to discuss a current illness or to practice preventive medicine. This culture is present focused and uses high-context communication, using few words. Eye contact is considered disrespectful; they are quiet, and frequently show little emotion. Medical professionals need to exercise care to avoid confusing these cultural traits with disinterest or defiant noncompliance. The primary caregiver is the extended family and may include members of their tribe.

Hispanic and Latino Cultures

People of Hispanic and Latino cultures are present focused, and accept Western medicine. However, they have an equally strong belief that the Christian God has control of their lives and that illness may be the result of sins against God. This can result in a fatalistic approach to treatment, or the idea that penance or other works on their part are required to cure an illness. As a result, the medical professional must be very careful in communicating treatment protocols and the importance of compliance. Showing respect by using direct eye contact is recommended to obtain cooperation in treatment. The extended family is involved in health care, with the mother or grandmother as principal caregiver.

 STOP AND CONSIDER

A Malaysian mother brings her 12-month old infant in for his annual physical examination.

1. How would the medical assistant go about discussing any cultural considerations with the mother before performing procedures?
2. How might the medical assistant explain the necessity of procedures and their relationship to growth and development patterns?
3. How will you demonstrate respect for this culture in your therapeutic communication?

Religion-Based Cultures

Religion can have as great an impact on communication in a medical setting as culture. People with a strong belief that their god will take care of all healing and who expect miraculous cures may be unwilling to allow themselves or their children to be treated by health care professionals. Those who believe in spiritualistic rituals and charms, or who rely on **folk medicine** prescribed by lay healers, may not follow the type of care prescribed in Western medicine. Still others will not allow the physician to do his or her job in diagnosing and treating an illness because the examination may violate a religious prohibition considered more important than life itself. Medical personnel involved with any of these groups must seek to identify the barriers to effective medical care and try to work within their framework to gain the confidence and respect of the client, so that therapeutic communication and treatment can result.

The key to overcoming barriers resulting from the religious convictions of clients is to understand their religious background. Being sensitive to the prohibitions and folk cures inherent in that religion or belief, and discussing with the client how they can be incorporated into treatment can overcome these barriers.

Judaism

Practitioners of Judaism worship on the Sabbath (from sunset Friday to sunset Saturday) versus Sunday for most Christians. They consider the Sabbath as a day of rest, and Orthodox Jews limit doing even such simple things as turning on a light switch or appliance. Scheduling medical tests or procedures on the Sabbath should first be discussed with the client.

Normal hospital routine is usually acceptable to people practicing Judaism, with the exception of dietary restrictions revolving around eating pork and food preparation techniques. **Kosher food** is available in most modern Western hospitals, but when it is not, vegetarian food and dairy products are frequently acceptable. During Passover, **leaven** is to be avoided. Judaism allows most tests and procedures as long as they preserve human life. Abortion is strictly prohibited. Mutilation of the body is forbidden, and this can cause some problem when an autopsy is required. It is allowed only when mandated by civil authorities. Judaism does not have special rituals involving dying clients, except that they should be attended by a chaplain or rabbi at the time of death.

Hinduism and Buddhism

Practitioners of Hinduism and Buddhism have similar religiously influenced cultural characteristics that can affect the medical practitioner. Both believe in reincarnation and hence are strict vegetarians. Buddhists may require meals be served before noon on special feast days. Buddhists may refuse pain medication that will prevent them from being mentally alert and aware. Most medical procedures that do not result in the destruction of life are acceptable. Modesty is important to both Hindus and Buddhists; consequently, short hospital or examination gowns will often be refused. Medical personnel of either sex are acceptable to all except priests. Priests are considered defiled if they touch or are touched by a woman.

Islam

The Islamic faith is frequently thought of as Middle Eastern or Arab; however, that is not true. The rapid growth of people embracing Islam throughout the world results in Muslims being found in almost every cultural **ethnic** group and country. All Arabs or people of Middle Eastern culture are not Muslim, however. People from this region are Muslim, Christian, or Jewish, with the majority being Muslim.

Embracing the Islamic faith radically changes the believer's inherent culture. The resulting modified culture differs significantly from their original culture. The male head of the household makes most decisions, even for a female client, and the immediate family is the primary caregiver. In some instances, it may be required that the male family members be told medical information prior to telling the client. Muslims are modest in dress, precluding a display of body parts; hospital or examination gowns are highly objectionable and many will refuse to wear them. Strict followers of Islam may not allow a female to be touched or examined by a male practitioner, and a woman who has never been married cannot have a pelvic examination due to concern that it may affect virginity. When a woman is examined, another person of the same sex must be present. Male Muslim clients may object to a female being in charge of their nursing care or as their physician.

Dietary requirements are part of Islamic-influenced culture. Non-pork or even a vegetarian diet may be followed, and alcohol is prohibited even as a base for medications. Daily prayers are part of the life of a strict Muslim, and not being allowed to follow this requirement can cause discomfort for a client. Ritual washing is a part of the preparation for prayer, as is washing private areas after using the toilet. The client's physical condition and availability of facilities will dictate the feasibility of compliance, but if at all possible the staff should comply with such requests to achieve the best recuperation and recovery from illness.

Miscellaneous cultural traits or taboo subjects exist in the Islamic faith that can interfere with medical treatment. Touching by people of the opposite sex is frowned upon, and shaking hands upon greeting is frequently not done even between men. Mental illness is not acceptable, and since birth defects are considered a test of their faith, they are frequently ignored and not discussed. Muslim clients are generally fatalistic and do not readily accept a terminal disease, because they believe that God controls all things. Hospice care is not usually acceptable to Muslims. These restrictions are only part of an extensive list of taboo subjects, and represent those that would be most likely to offend a person practicing Islam.

Table 2-2 summarizes the information regarding cultural and religious effects on health care presented in this section.

TABLE 2-2 Generalization of Cultural/Religious Effects on Health Care

Culture or Religion	Medical Care Background	Caregiving Structure	Communication Traits	Time Focus°
Caucasian, Western Culture	**Western Medicine**, rely on prescription medications, practice preventive medicine, may rely on holistic medicine or folk medicine in some rural areas.	**Individual**, immediate family, close friends.	**Low Context**, direct, eye contact expected, not adverse to therapeutic touching, may challenge medical opinions, basic English, speaks loudly.	**Future**
African American, Western Culture	**Western Medicine**, rely on prescription medications, practice preventive medicine, may rely on holistic medicine or folk medicine in some rural areas.	**Extended family**, relatives, close friends, neighbors, church family.	**Low Context**, direct, eye contact expected, not adverse to therapeutic touching, may challenge medical opinions and can distrust medical personnel, basic English sometimes mixed with street language (Ebonics).	**Present**/Future
Black, African, or Caribbean Culture	**Mixture** of Western and holistic medicine combined with spiritualism.	**Extended family**, relatives, close friends, neighbors, church family, tribal affiliation.	**Low Context**, eye contact expected, highly emotional, basic English strongly mixed with local dialect.	**Present**
Asian Culture Asian Indian, Chinese, Filipino, Japanese, Korean, Thai, Laotian, Vietnamese	**Mixture** of Western and holistic medicine combined with Confucian principals, i.e., mind control of the body and maintaining a balance between natural forces and energy in the body, eating foods designated as having hot and cold properties to cure illness is common, mental illness is considered shameful and is denied.	**Immediate family**, opinions of family and particularly elders are important.	**High Context**, indirect, avoid eye contact, show little emotion, avoid therapeutic touching, youth speak basic English, elders may speak little English, may agree with what is said even when they do not understand in order to avoid conflict or to avoid losing face, speak softly.	**Present**/Past
Native American, South Sea Island Cultures	**Mixture** of Western and folk medicine combined with importance of a balance between the forces of nature.	**Extended family**, relatives, close friends, neighbors, tribal affiliation.	**High Context**, avoid eye contact, speak softly and slowly. Basic English mixed with tribal dialects.	**Present**
Hispanic and Latino Cultures	**Mixture** of Western and folk medicine combined with a strong belief in intervention by God, eating foods designated as having hot and cold properties to cure illness is common. (See p. 49)	**Extended family**, relatives, church family, collective community.	**High Context**, be respectful and make direct eye contact, speak softly. Some basic English, most speak Spanish.	**Present**/Past

(continues)

TABLE 2-2   *(continued)*

Culture or Religion	Medical Care Background	Caregiving Structure	Communication Traits	Time Focus*
Judaism	**Western Medicine**, religion does not allow eating pork and requires kosher food.	Culturally dependent	Culturally dependent	**Future**/Present
Hinduism/Buddhism	**Western Medicine**, religions do not allow eating meat, modest regarding their body.	Culturally dependent	Culturally dependent	**Future**/Present
Islam	**Mixture** of Western and folk medicine combined with a strong belief in intervention by Allah. Match gender of caregiver and client. Woman may not be permitted to be examined by male medical professional, mental illness denied, do not ingest alcohol, believe complete rest is proper for all illnesses. Do not eat pork.	**Immediate family**, opinions of family and particularly male head of household are important	**High Context**, touching between men and women is prohibited for strict believers, do not discuss sexual dysfunction, females do not make direct eye contact, will not discuss many taboo subjects (mental illness, birth defects, contraception, hospice). Those from Middle East speak loudly to indicate the importance of what they are saying.	**Future**/Present

* stating that the bold term represents the predominent focus.

CULTURAL BROKERING

Cultural brokering is the act of bridging, linking, or mediating between groups or people through the process of reducing conflict or producing change (National Center for Cultural Competence, Georgetown University Center for Child and Human Development, Georgetown University Medical Center, 2004). A cultural broker may also be termed a cultural facilitator, or an interpreter who serves as a go-between, or one who advocates on behalf of another individual or group within the health care community. These individuals are trained professionals proficient in the knowledge and skills of cultural and medical language, and are employed in health care settings. Cultural brokers respect the values of diverse cultures and health care systems and are knowledgeable about both. They are able to overcome any existing language barriers, so that everyone understands each other clearly and mutual trust is fostered. They also have a working knowledge of possible community services for clients who may need support other than health care; examples include housing, food, clothing, child care, etc.

Using a Medical Interpreter/Broker

Federal laws enforced by the United States Department of Health and Human Services (DHHS) for the Office for Civil Rights (OCR) mandate the use of a trained interpreter/broker when clients cannot communicate because of language differences. The use of an interpreter/broker is especially helpful when consent forms are required, assessment questions are asked, and specific instructions are given to the client. Interviews of this nature require cultural sensitivity and an awareness of any legal and ethical implications. Using interpreters can increase the quality of care provided to clients. They aid the physician in acquiring a complete and accurate medical history to enable diagnosis of health care issues. When clients understand what is required for treatment, they are usually more compliant and will be willing to sign the necessary consent forms and follow treatment protocols.

Guidelines for using an interpreter/broker include the following:

- Brief the interpreter/broker. Discuss the reason for their presence and review the types of questions that may be asked during the interview and any goals to be achieved.

- Introduce the client and interpreter/broker and allow them some time to establish a rapport before the interview begins.

- Assure the client that confidentiality will be maintained and that nothing will be shared without the client's written permission to do so.

- During the interview, position yourself so that you can see both the interpreter/broker and the client, but maintain appropriate eye contact and direct questions to the client. Observe the client's nonverbal communication.

- Keep it short. Avoid long or complicated sentences during the interview. Focus on one subject at a time: i.e., *Do you have pain?* not *Do you have pain, tiredness or loss of appetite?*

- Do not interrupt during conversation between the client and interpreter/broker.

- Allow the interpreter/broker time to think. Do not be impatient.

- Be aware that the client may understand some English.

- Be sensitive to cultural diversity regarding age, gender, and socio-economic status between the client and the interpreter/broker. For example, selecting an interpreter who is of the same gender and similar age as the client may be helpful in some cultures. When working with Asian cultures, it may be wiser to choose an interpreter/broker who is older than the client and is viewed by the client as someone to be respected.

- Allow time with the interpreter/broker after the interview has been completed. This permits the interpreter to share anything that could not be shared in the client's presence, or to offer insight relating to impressions regarding nonverbal cues or culture preferences.

- Use the same interpreter/broker for any follow-up visits.

THE THERAPEUTIC RESPONSE

- If language is a significant barrier, consider using an interpreter/broker. See sections in this chapter, Cultural Brokering on p. 46 and Using a Medical Interpreter/Broker on p. 47.

- During the client interview, in addition to asking symptoms, ask the client what he or she thinks caused the illness and what treatment he or she thinks should be used to treat the illness. The client might also be asked how the illness was treated in the past.

- Do not belittle folk medicine or holistic treatments, and unless they are contra-indicated, consider allowing their continuation in order to develop the trust and respect of the client.

- Consider prescribing common folk treatments to achieve the medical results desired. An example would be prescribing healthful, cultural beverages such as a specific herbal tea to maintain hydration instead of simply prescribing water.

RECOGNIZING TYPES OF MEDICINE

Different cultures have evolved different approaches to understanding illnesses and problems with the human body. Western medicine is the only type of medicine that is based on the scientific method. That is not to say that other medicines are not effective. Most are based on past experience and rational theory, and in some cases, religious precepts. Understanding that a client has a background in other than Western medicine will assist Western medical personnel to better communicate with multicultural clients.

Ancient Greek Influence on Culture

The ancient Greeks may have had an influence on current **Oriental medicine**, and Hispanic folk medicine. The ancient Greeks believed that disease resulted from an imbalance in the **four humors**. All that remains of this concept today is a belief that disease results from an excess or deficiency of either hot or cold in either food or illnesses. Examples of hot diseases are hypertension, diabetes, stomach disorders, constipation, and insomnia. Examples of cold diseases are the common cold, menstrual cramps, diarrhea, and colic in infants. Hot disorders would be treated with cold foods or remedies, and vice versa. Examples of hot foods are potatoes, ginger, ice cream, fried foods, and high fat foods, whereas examples of cold foods are chicken, fish, fruit, boiled vegetables, and squash. Prescribing a diet that contradicts a client's cultural influences may result in the diet not being followed.

Western Medicine

Western medicine is based on the premise that disease results from bacterial and viral attack on the body. Diseases are diagnosed by observing the clients' symptoms and from scientific tests. Treatments consist of pharmaceutical products and surgical procedures, as appropriate. Mental state is recognized as contributing to wellness, but receives less consideration in most treatment regimes.

Holistic Medicine

Holistic medicine focuses on 1) personal accountability for one's health; 2) the human body's ability to heal itself; and 3) balancing the body, mind, and spirit with the environment. It is known by terms that include accommodative, integrative, complementary, alternative, or natural medicine. Holistic medicine encompasses acupuncture, biofeedback, chiropractic, folk medicine, meditation, megavitamin therapy, spiritual healing, yoga, and others. This approach to health recognizes the client as a whole person, not just a disease or a collection of symptoms.

Oriental Medicine

The objective of **Oriental medicine** is to restore balance between energy states within the body to provide movement, to act as a defense against pathological agents, and to promote physical growth. A balance between opposing states is paramount in Oriental medicine. Cold versus hot, interior versus exterior, and deficiency versus excess are examples of opposing states. Foods we eat, our state of mind, and environmental conditions all interact to maintain a balance. Oriental medicine treats illness using acupuncture, massage, herbal medicine, meditation, and exercise and may be considered a subset of alternative medicine.

Folk Medicine

Folk medicine employs home remedy medications without a scientific understanding of the processes involved, and usually has been handed down from earlier times. For example, the wormwood plant has been used to treat fevers in China for 2,000 years. Recently a compound found in the wormwood plant has been used in a new antimalarial drug. The Hispanic culture uses chili peppers to treat pain. Today pharmaceutical companies utilize capsaicin as a topical cream for arthritis pain. Many folk medicines are beneficial, or at least do not cause harmful effects; others however, are considered dangerous. An example of a dangerous drug is *azarcón* or *greta*. It is used to treat stomach ailments in Guatemala. The drug contains lead and is known to cause seizures, coma, and even death. Another example is *kava kava*, an herb used by Pacific Islanders to make an anxiety-relieving tea. Drinking a concentrated form of this tea poisons the liver.

Folk healers practice in their homes, or in a religious setting. There are many names given to these healers. Examples include grannies and herbalists, whose learning has been primarily passed down from generation to generation. Spiritual healers describe receiving their gift during profound religious experiences. They are more likely to use prayer, laying on of hands, and holy oil or water with supernatural powers to heal. Supernatural healers may be referred to as sorcerers, voodooists, or root doctors.

Clients who take folk medicine may not readily share this information with their health care professionals. Therefore, it is important to listen carefully when taking the client history, observe the client carefully without being judgmental, and ask questions about the illness and any remedies or treatments they may have tried. Clients involved in folk medicine often wear charms, **amulets**, or copper or silver bracelets believed to protect or warn of illness.

Summary

Learning more about cultural diversity is a very enriching experience. Each culture is unique; each is good; one is not better than another; one may be more familiar to us, but that does not make it better. It is important to practice techniques that build and foster multicultural therapeutic communication. This involves learning about the beliefs and values of different cultures and religions and recognizing any barriers, including biases or prejudices that may impact multicultural therapeutic communicaiton. Using a cultural brokering service or interpreter who is able to interpret the client's language and specific cultural nuances, as well as the health care culture's terminology, aids the medical team in providing the best health care. When possible, consider allowing any procedures or alternative treatments that are comforting to the client and that are not detrimental to the treatment regimen being prescribed.

EXERCISES

Exercise 1

First, turn to the glossary and review the meaning of *bias* and *prejudice*. Using the columns provided, list cultures and then the biases and prejudices you recognize in yourself when communicating with diverse cultures.

Culture	Biases	Prejudices

What steps might you initiate to decrease these biases and prejudices?

Exercise 2

Using the following questions, assess your own cultural background, recognizing that cultural values are principles or standards that members of a cultural group share in common. Each background will have both shared values and individualized values.

1. Identify your culture.
2. List three cultural values that your culture possesses.
3. List three cultural values that are important to you as an individual.
4. Discuss how these personal values directly relate to your culture's attitudes, beliefs, and behaviors.
5. Discuss how your cultural values have influenced the way in which others perceive and react to you.
6. Using the Internet and your favorite search engine, investigate a culture that you are not familiar with. Print out pages related to this culture and discuss similarities and differences between various cultures with a classmate.

Exercise 3

Visit a market in an ethnic neighborhood.

1. Describe the market.

2. Were you familiar with any of the foods or items sold in this market?

3. Describe the shoppers and the sales personnel in this market. How did they interact and communicate?

4. What was your comfort level while in the market?

5. Do you find or observe any biases toward *you*?

   Visualize the market as a health care facility, with you as the client and the sales personnel representing health care professionals.

6. What could the market sales personnel have done to make you feel more comfortable?

7. From the marketplace experience, develop a written plan of what you could do in a health care setting to make the experience more comfortable for a person of another culture.

REVIEW QUESTIONS

Multiple Choice

1. Three important factors to consider when developing multicultural therapeutic communication include

   a. learning about the beliefs and values of different cultures, practicing using barriers to cultural communication, and participating in discussions with multicultural individuals.

   b. determining your own cultural beliefs, practicing using barriers to cultural communication, and participating in discussions with multicultural individuals.

   c. learning about the beliefs and values of different cultures, recognizing any barriers to cultural communication, and practicing techniques that build and foster multicultural communication.

   d. determining your own cultural beliefs, practicing techniques that build and foster multicultural communication, and participating in discussions with multicultural individuals.

2. A high-context communication style involves *all* of the following *except* that it

   a. relies mainly on explicit and highly detailed language.

   b. involves great reliance on body language as a communicator.

   c. references objects in the environment.

   d. uses culturally relevant phraseology to convey an idea.

3. All of the statements regarding present-oriented individuals are true *except* that

   a. in the past they struggled daily with meeting basic needs.

   b. cultures where basic needs are naturally provided in abundance tend to be present-oriented.

   c. present-oriented individuals do not look on time as being important and tend to be careless about promptness.

   d. present-oriented individuals see time as circular or continuous and repeating.

4. Ethnocentrism means

   a. a slant toward a particular belief.

   b. the belief that one's own culture and traditions are better than those of others.

   c. an opinion or judgment that is formed before all the facts are known.

   d. usually a preconceived and unfavorable concept.

5. The ideal interpreter will be able to do all of the following *except*

   a. interpret the client's language.

   b. interpret the client's specific cultural nuances.

   c. interpret an equivalent meaning of the client's response.

   d. mandates the use of trained interpreters.

FOR FURTHER CONSIDERATION

1. How can you, as a health care professional, recognize the uniqueness of each culture, including your own, and incorporate this uniqueness into therapeutic communication?

2. When language is a communication barrier, how might the health care facility take steps to ensure that therapeutic communication is possible?

3. Preconceived negative biases or prejudices about clients of different cultures hamper therapeutic relationships. How might the health care professional assess personal negative biases or prejudices?

CASE STUDIES

Case Study 1

A health care professional attempted to explain infant care techniques to Iranian parents. Since the mother was not feeling well, the health care professional began explaining everything to the husband. He refused to listen, stating that in his country, men did not get involved in child care.

1. Using information from this chapter and research through the Internet, investigate cultural values and beliefs of Middle Eastern families. The American Journal of Obstetrics & Gynecology's Web site provides a beginning for your search (http://www.ajog.org).

2. What therapeutic communication techniques would be appropriate in this situation?

Case Study 2

Mr. Suzuki, a Japanese man in his seventies, recently experienced a stroke that resulted in right-side weakness. He spent several weeks in a rehabilitation center relearning self-care activities and tasks involved in daily living. His therapist spent a great deal of time with Mr. Suzuki and his family, explaining through practical instruction how these skills could be accomplished. Mr. Suzuki and his wife sat passively through the instructions.

During the therapy sessions with staff members, Mr. Suzuki was compliant and made good progress in relearning self-care activities, and was able to walk using a walker. When Mr. Suzuki was back in his room, he expected his wife to do everything for him, even self-care activities that he did for himself during therapy sessions.

1. Use the Internet to learn more about Japanese values and beliefs regarding health care and family.

2. Identify the cultural characteristics that may be potential problems in Mr. Suzuki's rehabilitation.

3. What actions can be taken to minimize the impact of these cultural characteristics?

Resources

Galanti, G. (2004). *Caring for patients of different cultures* (3rd ed.). Philadelphia, PA: University of Pennsylvania Press.

Hammoud, M. M., White, C. B., & Fetters, M. D. (2005). Opening cultural doors: providing culturally sensitive healthcare to Arab American and American Muslim patients. *American Journal of Obstetrics and Gynecology. 193*(4), 1307–1311.

LaVeist, T. A., Nickerson, K. J., & Bowie, J. V. (2000). Attitudes about racism, medical mistrust, and satisfaction with care among African American and white cardiac patients. *Medical Care Research and Review, 57*(Supplement 1), 146–161.

Lindh, W. Q., Pooler, M. S., Tamparo, C. D., & Dahl, B. M. (2006). *Comprehensive medical assisting: administrative and clinical competencies* (3rd ed.). Albany, NY: Thomson Delmar Learning.

Luckmann, J. (2000). *Transcultural communication in health care.* Albany, NY: Thomson Delmar Learning.

National Center for Cultural Competence (Spring/Summer 2004). *Bridging the cultural divide in health care settings: The essential role of cultural broker programs.* Georgetown University Center for Child and Human Development; Georgetown University Medical Center. Washington, DC.

Purnell, L. D., & Paulanka, B. J. (2003). *Transcultural health care: a culturally competent approach* (2nd ed.). Philadelphia, PA: F.A. Davis Company.

Purnell, L. D., & Paulanka, B. J. (2005). *Guide to culturally competent health care.* Philadelphia, PA: F.A. Davis Company.

Salimbene, S. (2000). *What language does your patient hurt in?* St. Paul, MN: EMCParadigm.

Wurtz, E. (2005). A cross-cultural analysis of websites from high-context cultures and low-context cultures. http://jcmc.indiana.edu/vol11/issue1/wuertz.html

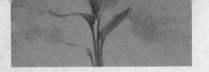

CHAPTER
3

THE HELPING INTERVIEW

CHAPTER OBJECTIVES

The learner should strive to meet the following chapter objectives and demonstrate an understanding of the facts and principles presented in this chapter through written and oral communication.

- Define key term as presented in the glossary.
- Identify the purpose of the helping interview.
- Identify the three primary components of the helping interview.
- List and contrast the feelings experienced by the individual giving help and the individual needing help.
- Identify a minimum of 10 important preparations to be made by the health care professional before the interview takes place.
- Describe the following attributes and their use in the helping interview.
  - risk/trust
  - warmth/caring
  - genuineness
  - sympathy/empathy
  - sincerity
- Describe the following responding skills and their use.
  - sharing observations
  - acknowledging feelings

- clarifying and validating
- reflecting and paraphrasing
- Discuss the *levels of need* and relate them to the helping interview.
- Define the following and differentiate how they encourage or discourage the therapeutic exchange.
  - closed questions
  - open questions
  - indirect statements
- Describe the following blocks to therapeutic communication.
  - reassuring clichés/stereotypical comments
  - giving advice/approval
  - requesting/requiring an explanation
  - belittling
  - defending
  - changing the subject/shifting
- Demonstrate or list the steps involved in an appropriate closure of a helping interview.

OPENING CASE STUDY

James Alonzo is on his way to his doctor's office. He has no desire to do this. His wife made him come for a physical exam. It has been five years since his last one. He rarely sees the doctor. James had to take a couple of hours off work in the middle of a really busy project to keep his appointment. He steps into the clinic, up to the front desk, and gives his name. The receptionist asks for his insurance card and tells him to be seated. He wonders how long he will have to wait as he picks up a magazine. He says to himself, "The atmosphere in this place is about like the drive-up window for fast food."

After 20 minutes, a young woman comes to the doorway and calls out his name. He follows her down the hallway. She stops in front of the scale and asks him to step up. She jots the weight in his chart and takes him into the examination room. The conversation continues.

"So, I see you have come for a physical exam today."

"Yeah. My wife made me come, even made the appointment."

"Are you having any symptoms today? Are you taking any medications?"

"I take an aspirin occasionally, and antacids."

"How often do you take the antacids?"

"Oh, I keep them in my pocket, maybe once a day or so."

James kind of wants to talk to the doctor about having difficulty emptying his bladder, but he is not about to tell this woman this, especially when she looks as young as his high-school-aged daughter.

"I am going to take your blood pressure now. Please remove your shirt."

James removes his shirt and puts it on his lap. When the assistant is finished, she tells James to take off all his clothes and put on the gown. The doctor will be in shortly. James removes his clothes, but doesn't know what to do with his underwear, and wonders if he should leave his socks on. He waits another 10 minutes before the doctor comes in.

"Good afternoon, James. What brings you in?"

"My wife says it is past time for me to have a physical."

"Let's see. It has been quite a while since you were in. You are 58 now, right? Your weight is up about 15 pounds, I see, and your blood pressure is somewhat elevated. We better address the antacids you are taking, too. Any problems you want to share with me?"

"Well, I kind of want to ask you about a problem I have when I pee. I can't seem to get it all out, and I have to go quite often. It is kind of embarrassing when I am standing in a public restroom at the urinal and everyone is done before I am."

"You might have an enlarged prostate. I'll know better after I examine you." As the doctor starts to listen to James's chest sounds, James begins to sweat. He is thinking, "Oh no! Prostate! If he has to do anything about that, I won't be any good at sex anymore."

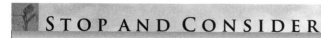

STOP AND CONSIDER

1. In what ways did the opening case scenario encourage communication?
2. What things will the doctor focus on?
3. Will all of James's concerns be addressed?
4. What would you have done differently?

INTRODUCTION

Seeking care in any type of health care facility is usually not the most favorite activity of any individual. It is likely viewed as a "necessary evil," something that must be done but is not pleasantly anticipated. Making the encounter between health care professional and client both helpful and therapeutic is a challenge. The techniques in this chapter will help to facilitate therapeutic communications between health care professionals and clients.

CHANGES IN TODAY'S HEALTH CARE CLIMATE

A large number of clients seeking care in today's health care climate come with far more information than ever before experienced in medicine. Consumers are bombarded daily by advertisements touting the claims of the latest medicines that are sure to cure the worst of ills and informing them of any and all possible side effects. Consumers already taking the prescribed medicine can become alarmed by the warnings given in the media; others, fearing they suffer from the described malady, are anxious to tell their doctors they want that medication.

Consumers are likely to conduct a fair amount of independent research via the Internet prior to seeking a physician's advice or accepting their physician's diagnosis or treatment plan. A second opinion is quite accessible, and in many instances no longer needs a recommendation from your doctor or insurance approval. Some physicians are concerned about the accuracy and validity of information found on the Internet. Clients seeking medical information via the Internet must realize that such information is not specific to their particular case and does not take into account the same personal information their primary care physician has about them. While the vastness of the Internet may not provide the best information at all times, many consumers find it more friendly and nonthreatening than their physician's clinic and staff. There are even sites on the Internet to assist clients in making medical choices.

Consumers also may find their continuity of care interrupted by their employer's choices of health care plans, which can force a change in providers. For many, having the same physician for a decade or more is increasingly uncommon. It becomes progressively more difficult to ensure that clients' complete health care records are in the hands of their current provider, even with the use of electronic medical records.

One of the most important aspects of the helping interview is empowering clients to become equal partners in their health care. The successful interview will help clients focus on their needs and encourage open and free "give-and-take" communication with their primary provider. A closer look at the components of the helping interview and how to make it a successful encounter for both the client and the health care provider will help consumers receive the best possible medical care.

INTERVIEW COMPONENTS

A *helping interview* is a conversation between a health care professional and a person in need and is a common tool of communication in any health care setting. Three components of the helping interview are

1. The *orientation* of the professional and the client to each other

2. The *identification* of the client's problem

3. The *resolution* of the client's problem

The helping interview is usually planned for a set time and place, with the health care professional in control. It is this control that often intimidates clients.

Control Factor

Control is a critical factor in the helping interview, but should not be abused. Even the use of the word *patient* implies a superior/inferior, higher/lower, more-knowledge/less-knowledge relationship. The helping interview clearly involves people in an unequal partnership. Being in a state of need or helplessness is not empowering. Consider the following feelings likely to describe giving and needing help.

Giving Help Feels	Needing Help Feels
Important	Unimportant or inadequate
Useful	Useless or depressed
Powerful	Powerless
Gratified	Frightened or embarrassed
Happy	Sad or angry

It is more pleasant to give help than to need help. Health care professionals must be constantly aware of how their status affects persons seeking help. Clients should be empowered as much as possible by the experience in the helping interview, since empowered clients are likely to participate more fully in their care and return to health faster (Figure 3-1).

Orientation

There are some important preparations to be made by the health care professional even before the interview takes place. Personal appearance and the appearance of the medical facility or examination room are vital keys to getting the helping interview off to a good start.

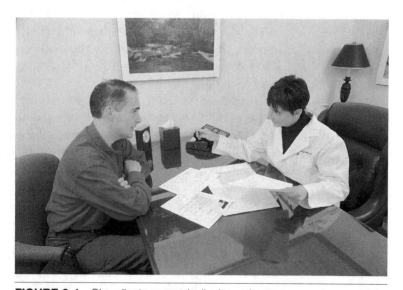

FIGURE 3-1 Give clients as much dignity and empowerment as possible.

Comprehensive Medical Assisting Administrative & Clinical Competencies, W. Lindh, M. Pooler, C. Tamparo, J. Cerrato, Delmar Publishers, Albany NY 1998.

Personal appearance and grooming must be professional and impeccable. The health care professional, always alert to the control of any disease-producing organisms, will remember that personal cleanliness helps reduce pathogens and inhibits their transmission.

The client expects a health care professional to look and dress the part. In fact, the client may have difficulty trusting someone who is too casual in appearance. A name tag that includes your title and credential is most helpful.

Consider the facility's surroundings and the examination room. Will the setting encourage an equal relationship? Are you seated near the client or with a desk between you? Is the examination room so small that the client must sit on the examination table? If possible, be seated facing the client and at the same level. The client should not, if at all possible, be disrobed during the orientation phase of the interview.

Greet your client in a pleasant manner and with a name when possible. Even in a busy clinic with a number of waiting clients in the reception area, it is not too difficult to identify the next client to be seen. Check the chart carefully to make certain it matches the client you are about to approach. Step close to the client to preserve confidentiality as you begin the helping interview. "Mr. Alonzo? Please come with me." Some clients bring another person with them, to accompany them during the actual examination. If this is the case, accommodations must be made for that individual. As you escort the client to the examination area, observe mobility and alertness. Always match your pace to the client's, so he/she does not feel left behind, and offer any assistance that might be needed. Making "small talk" as you walk, you might comment: "I apologize for your wait; we got a little backed up today." Or, "Did you have trouble parking?"

Introduce yourself and give your title, as the client may not know it. Be certain to get the client's name and pronounce it correctly. Do not address the client informally unless the client requests that you do so. If the interview is conducted in the examination room, knock before entering.

Speak with a comfortable and appropriate tone and voice volume. Do not speak in a monotone. Make certain the client hears and understands you. If there is a language barrier or speech problem, get an expert to help you. Do not try to speak a language of which you really have only a little knowledge. Time is an important element; the health care professional must have time to hear the client. The helping interview is no place for misunderstanding.

Risk/Trust

As the interview gets underway, be aware that the conversation involves a fair amount of risk on the part of the client. The health care professional needs to build an atmosphere of trust, making the risk easier. As the trust level increases, it is easier for the client to share feelings and attitudes about the problem. Trust has to be earned. Without it, the helping relationship will go no further than mere introductions. The health care professional is responsible for nurturing mutual trust.

Warmth/Caring

Warmth may be defined as an attitude expressing caring and concern. It is primarily communicated through facial expressions, such as a caring look or smile, that cross all cultural differences. A calm, reassuring voice also expresses warmth and caring. Another expression of caring and warmth comes from the health care professional who gives full attention to the client and what is being said. Clients who sense that they are the most important person to the health care professional at that time are more likely to relax in a nonthreatening atmosphere where they feel free to express concerns. Caring expresses a liking or regard for others, and communicates a watchfulness for cues that may indicate the problem and its possible solution.

Genuineness

Genuineness is being real and honest with others. The health care professional must be able to communicate honestly with others while being careful not to judge or condemn. Genuineness assures there will be congruency between the verbal and nonverbal messages. Genuineness and acceptance are partners in the helping interview.

Sympathy/Empathy

To show *sympathy* is to respond to the emotional state of others and to acknowledge the feelings expressed by clients. Sympathy states, "I am available to you." *Empathy* is the ability to accept another's private world as if it were your own. It is fair and sensitive; it is an awareness of others' situations and what they are experiencing. It communicates identification with and understanding of another's situation. Empathy states, "I'm available to walk this road with you." Expressing sympathy and/or empathy encourages clients to express their concerns and helps them cope. The most therapeutic health care providers recognize that when they listen sympathetically to their clients, clients are better able to recognize their own completeness and strength.

Sincerity

Sincerity involves those attributes already identified, as well as creating an atmosphere that is free from hypocrisy. The sincere health care professional is forthright, candid, and truthful. Health care professionals must be sincere in their intentions and communications with others. Sincerity cannot be faked. If clients do not believe in your sincerity, they may "shut down."

IDENTIFICATION OF PROBLEM

Once the orientation phase has been completed and the trust level is fairly well established, it is time to turn attention to the problem or problems identified by the client. As well as remembering to listen with the "third ear," (that is, being aware of what the client is *not* saying or picking up on hints as to the real message), there are a number of techniques that will ease the communication between clients and health care professionals. These techniques may be referred to as *responding skills*, and are identified in the next section.

Responding Skills

There are a number of skills for the health care professional to keep in mind during the helping interview.

Sharing Observations

Observations will focus on both the client's physical and emotional state. The statement "You seem upset" conveys concern and interest in knowing more, and comes from the health care professional's observation of the client. The tone of voice, eye contact, and body position are all factors to be considered in observations. Statements such as "You are trembling" or "You seem to be in pain" are examples of shared observations. Such statements encourage the client to verbalize their feelings.

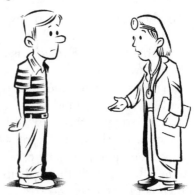

"YOU SEEM TO BE IN PAIN."

Acknowledging Feelings

Sharing observations is a way to acknowledge the client's feelings. This responding skill communicates to clients that their feelings are understood and accepted. It encourages verbalization by providing a safe, nonthreatening environment. An example of such an acknowledgment is "I know not sleeping at night because of the cough is distressing." Such acknowledgment makes it easier for clients to reveal their symptoms.

Clarifying and Validating

Clarifying is used when the health care professional is not certain of the meaning of the message communicated. Such statements as "I'm not sure I understand what you mean" or "Do you mean…?" are examples of clarification. Words used during an exchange may hold different meanings for others, so clarifying is important. This is especially critical when languages are different or may be easily misunderstood. For the message to be therapeutic, both parties must understand the same meaning and use the terms in the same manner.

Reflecting and Paraphrasing

Reflecting focuses on the emotional aspect of the client's expression. It involves listening to the verbal message as well as considering the nonverbal cues being sent. Facial expression and tone of voice will provide insight regarding the meaning of the message and its congruency. When using reflecting skills, "You feel" will often be used at the beginning of or within the response: for example, "You feel like the medicine is not helping."

Paraphrasing simply restates in the professional's own words what the client said. Its focus is more on the cognitive aspects of the message than on the feelings. Paraphrasing allows the client to hear what was just said and to verify the accuracy of the professional's listening ability. It is often helpful to tie together reflecting and paraphrasing. Using words such as "You feel…because…" connects the two skills easily: for example, "You feel the medicine is not helping because you still have the headaches."

LEVELS OF NEED

Paul Welter, in *How to Help a Friend*, identifies the helping relationship and levels of need. To become an effective helper, it is necessary to recognize what level of need your client has. Although this chart was

TABLE 3-1 Levels of Need

Level and Definition	Characteristics of Person in Need	Effective Helping Response
Problem		
Has a solution.	Asks specific question; wants immediate advice or information.	Supply information or advice.
Predicament		
No easy solution.	Often feels trapped; is not helped by advice.	The helper gets involved; works for openness.
Crisis		
A very large predicament; short-term.	Has a sense of urgency; may want help but is afraid to ask.	Expects you to help; bring client into present; accept emotions.
Panic		
A state of fear; sees only one way out.	Does not listen; mind is caught in dreadful future event; nonrational.	Move client from panic to "hold"; use touch; eye contact.
Shock		
A numbed or dazed condition.	Fails to take action; mind lapses for short time; unable to recall lapse.	Must act for this person. Stay with this person until back to normal.

established for helping friends, much of it can be adapted to recognizing the needs of clients who come for help. See Table 3-1, Levels of Need.

The Appendix A (see p. 224) provides a section related to Abraham Maslow, who developed criteria for determining a person's needs. He believed that individuals move back and forth from one need to another, depending upon their circumstances. Clients seeking treatment for medical problems are likely to be experiencing both physiologic and safety needs.

Recognizing that clients have different levels of need helps professionals to focus their attention correctly. Keeping in mind the attributes identified and the levels of need creates an atmosphere in which clients can ask questions that will assist them in fully identifying the problems they face.

QUESTIONING TECHNIQUES

Real skill is involved in knowing how to ask questions in a manner that helps the client express problems. These questions and answers are important to the identification and resolution of the problem. Also, they become the foundation for the client's medical record. There are three major types of questions that are useful during the helping interview, and each has its own appropriateness.

Closed Questions

Closed questions are useful in collecting information during the client history, and are most common at the beginning of the verbal exchange. They do not require the individual being asked the question to enlarge upon the answer. The questions usually begin with *do, is,* or *are,* and are answered with a simple *yes, no,* or a brief phrase. Examples of closed questions are

"Are you experiencing pain now?"

"Does it hurt when you raise your arm?"

"Is the bandage too tight?"

Open-Ended Questions

Open-ended questions are most helpful for therapeutic communication, as they encourage clients to identify more of the problem. They do not put words into clients' mouths; rather they allow clients to express their own thoughts and feelings. Open-ended questions usually begin with *how, what,* or *could.* They are an invitation for clients to express more detail. Examples of open-ended questions are

"Could your new job be responsible for a change in your eating habits?"

"What foods seem to trigger the need for antacids?"

"What did the doctor tell you about this medication?"

Indirect Statements

Open-ended questions can be reworded so that they become indirect statements. Indirect statements call for a response from the client, but do not make the client feel like he/she is being questioned. They do, however, encourage verbalization and express interest in the client from the health care professional. Examples of indirect statements are

"I'd like to hear about your new therapy program."

"Tell me what worries you most about this problem."

During the helping interview, it is beneficial to stay away from the use of questions that begin with *why*. When questions begin with *why*, clients often become defensive or feel they are being accused. Questions beginning with *how* or *what* are much more effective. This and other roadblocks to communication are identified in the next section.

Roadblocks to Communication

There are so many roadblocks to communication that one marvels at how *any* communication is effective. In therapeutic communication, preventing roadblocks is vital to a quality relationship with the client.

Some of the most common roadblocks to therapeutic communication are

reassuring clichés

giving advice/approval

requiring explanations

belittling/contradicting/criticizing

defending

changing subject/shifting

moralizing/lecturing

shaming/threatening/ridiculing

Health care professionals must keep in mind that when clients seek care for some problem or ailment, they have delicate psychological and mental attitudes and must be handled with care, to put them at ease. It also must be remembered that every communication is a transcultural one. Therefore, paying close attention to communication roadblocks is vital.

Reassuring Clichés

Reassuring **clichés** are often given automatically, and consist of patterned responses; trite expressions; or empty, meaningless phrases that express false assumptions about how a client feels. When the health care professional senses the client may be anxious or stressed, reassuring clichés may be expressed in an effort to reduce these feelings. However, the client will likely interpret clichés to mean the professional does not understand the problem or is not interested in becoming involved. These phrases also may be used by health care professionals to reduce their own personal anxieties. Examples of reassuring clichés are

"Everything will be all right."

"Keep your chin up. Hang in there."

Giving Advice/Approval

Giving advice may occur when health care professionals act from a subconscious desire to have all the answers, or feel the need to control the client's thoughts or actions. This usually occurs when the health care professional is doing more talking than listening. When clients are told what they should do, opinions and solutions are imposed on them. This advice-giving usually begins with "If I were you…" or "You should…" Recognition of the fact that these phrases are being used should trigger a warning signal to stop. No one can ever be in the exact circumstances or situations of another person. Remember, the goal is to sufficiently empower the client, who will then be able to recognize what advice might be needed. Even when the physician gives directions to clients, the phrase used should be "My recommendation is…"

Requiring Explanations

Asking clients to explain their reasons for feelings, behaviors, or thoughts requires them to analyze and explain these experiences. Questions that ask *why* are intimidating. Examples include "Why do you think you are feeling that way?" and "Why did you do that?" Often clients may not understand the reasons for the discomfort to begin with. They may understand the discomfort but not know how to describe it, or they may not have sufficient trust in the health care professional to risk sharing their feelings. During the helping interview, health care professionals should ask clients to describe their feelings rather than explain them. This approach is nonthreatening and communicates to clients that their feelings are acceptable. It encourages clients to continue describing their situation.

Belittling/Contradicting/Criticizing

Expressions such as "You couldn't have bled that much" or "You shouldn't feel that way" send a message to the client: "You are mistaken; your feelings are unimportant." When a client comes with a concern or a

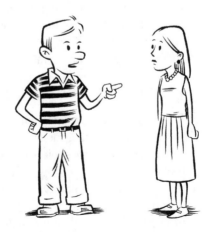

"YOU SHOULDN'T FEEL THAT WAY."

complaint, responding negatively will close the communication process immediately. The client feels what the client feels. Even if the professional knows that what is being described is impossible, clients are still the only ones who know their own body and feelings. Listen to and acknowledge the client's statements. Do not contradict.

There is *never* any time in a therapeutic relationship when a client should be criticized. Even if a client does something that is foolish, harmful, and extremely unhealthy, criticism does not open the lines of communication for wise, safe, and healthy advice or information.

Defending

"No one in this clinic would tell you that." When the health care professional defends something or someone the client has criticized, it implies the client has no right to express his/her feelings, concerns, or impressions. This contradiction will block the therapeutic exchange and prevent further verbalization by the client.

Changing the Subject/Shifting

When the health care professional changes the subject or shifts to new topics, the direction of the conversation will be controlled by the professional rather than allowing clients to discuss freely what they choose. Shifting the trust of the helping interview toward the health care professional's perceptions also blocks the exchange. Once the client has been blocked, he/she may discontinue future attempts to share feelings, concerns, or problems. Examples of changing the subject or shifting are

Client: "I will not have any more chemotherapy."

Professional: "Did your daughter visit this week?"

The professional might change the subject because he/she is uncomfortable with the topic or simply may want to gain information related to another specific subject. Care should be used in changing the subject or shifting to a new topic, to be certain it is appropriate to the present verbal exchange.

Moralizing/Lecturing

Health care professionals who easily criticize probably moralize also. Even though the client appears with a condition caused by a lifestyle that is totally contrary to society's standards of health, expressing judgment is unlikely to have a positive effect on the client. To moralize is to be unable to fully and completely accept the client's needs. In Elaine's situation, described in Chapter 1, her self-esteem was partly preserved by the refusal of her health care professionals to moralize over her decision. Health care professionals who work daily with substance-abuse addicts must not moralize, but must be able to see the person who was or who can be again.

Health care professionals, with all their knowledge and many years of experience, are apt to lecture. They might feel the lecture is quite appropriate to the situation, but even when the sharing of information is vital to the client's well-being, to lecture only makes the client feel defensive or of little value.

Shaming/Threatening/Ridiculing

To ridicule or shame a client will close communication immediately. Most often, this ridicule or shame is in the form of nonverbal rather than verbal communication. Health care professionals have been taught not to ridicule or shame, but these behaviors often show in actions rather than words. To laugh at a client's description of an ailment or misunderstanding of basic body functions is a common example of ridicule. To threaten a client with the consequences of some act only causes fear, submission, and resentment. It does nothing to encourage the client to change behavior. Clients are able to determine for themselves if their actions are damaging and what the consequences will be. Health care professionals who threaten are usually insecure or feel total responsibility for their clients. Neither characteristic is healthy.

RESOLUTION OF THE PROBLEM

As the helping interview nears completion, a couple of questions can be asked to make certain that clients have had the opportunity to express all their concerns. These questions might be "Is there anything else you would like to ask me today?" "Are there any other concerns that you have?" As the helping interview comes to a close, it is hoped that some resolution of the problem is also obvious. While many problems will require ongoing care, there should be some problem resolution in each helping interview. It is important for the health care professional to use the clearest and simplest language possible, since most clients have little or no knowledge of medical terminology. It is important to remember this: if the receiver has not understood the message as it was sent, no communication has taken place.

Most clients seek an explanation for their problem, and want to know how the resolution of the problem is going to affect their lives, how much time to allow for this resolution, and what future impact the problem may have. For example, a client who has been diagnosed with ulcerative colitis might be told, "Mr. Olson, the results of all our tests show that you have ulcerative colitis. We do not understand the cause of this illness, but there are no indications that any serious damage has occurred at this time. With proper treatment and medication, we should be able to keep active flare-ups at a minimum and prevent further complications."

The interview might continue at this point with a discussion of the client's lifestyle. Continue the discussion with ways to help the client cope with the impact of this disease and a description of the treatment necessary. It might also continue as follows: "There is no cure for this disease and you may have many exacerbations and remissions throughout your life, but if this treatment works, there should be no complicating medical problems. However, it is important for us to treat this problem now, because untreated, it can become serious. It is a good idea for you to include more fiber in your diet. I have a suggested nutritional plan here for you to consider. If certain foods cause diarrhea, then eliminate them from your diet or do not eat them during an active flare-up. In the active stage of this disease, avoid excess stress as much as possible. Also, I have a prescription to give you to assist the healing process in your lower colon, and medication to help prevent complications. You should see an improvement within several days."

Allow time for the client to think about what has just been said and to formulate any questions that arise. This is a good time to fill out the prescription or to get the nutritional guidelines from your file. Even saying "You must have some questions now, too" can be helpful to the client. If there are no questions at this point, remind the client, "Remember to call me any time you have a question. If you have any concerns or you are not better in a few days, call me. I will want to see you again in six weeks to make certain that we are on the right track."

It is most helpful to write out instructions for clients or to provide them with some written material explaining the procedures they are to follow. The best medical advice can be lost if clients do not correctly follow instructions.

It cannot be emphasized enough that the helping interview will either be the key to a health care professional's success or the end of what might have been a therapeutic relationship. Recall the incident identified in Chapter 1 (see p. 2) with Mrs. Nelson, who had been seriously injured by the dog. Consider how different the outcome might have been had her primary care physician been more "in tune" with her needs during the interview.

CASE STUDY

When Mrs. Nelson called her primary care physician, it would have been much more therapeutic had the assistant said, "Oh, Mrs. Nelson, how awful. You say the emergency room physician asked that you have a blood test this morning and that you have his records with you? We usually only see patients receiving complete physicals in the morning, but I believe that

continues

Case Study continued

the doctor will want to comply with the emergency room physician. Would you mind if you had to wait a bit when you come in?"

Mrs. Nelson, who has already shown that she is a compliant client, responds in the affirmative and the assistant selects a time where the wait will be as minimal as possible. When she is ushered into the examination room with her physician and the blood has been taken, the doctor might have said, "My assistant tells me you had a frightening experience with a dog, Mrs. Nelson. Tell me what happened."

While the doctor listens and observes Mrs. Nelson, he will notice her bandaged head and finger and how uncomfortable she appears. It is likely that questions will be asked of Mrs. Nelson regarding the medical chart from the emergency room to further enhance her physician's record. It seems important, also, for the doctor to say, "May I remove your bandage to have a look at your injury while the assistant is checking your blood count for us?"

Both head and finger wounds are examined and appropriately bandaged by the doctor. Throughout this process, and a discussion of the fractured tailbone and ways to be more comfortable, Mrs. Nelson is still showing anxiety. The doctor might then say,

"You seem quite anxious and worried, Mrs. Nelson."

"Well, I am, I guess. This is a heck of a spot to be in. I love dogs so much; to think I could be attacked by one! If I lose my little poodle, I will be really mad. And you know, my husband and I are about to celebrate our 52nd wedding anniversary. We usually go someplace. I guess I won't be doing that, will I?"

"It is pretty hard to see a dog attack your dog and get hurt in the meantime, I know. I have a dog, and I think I would feel awful if something like that happened to her, especially when she did nothing to provoke the attack. How is your poodle?"

"Well, the vet says he will make it, but he looks awful. My husband picked him up at the vet this morning."

"As for going somewhere, you should still be able to go. You can remove this bandage tomorrow and come back in two days so I can remove the stitches. Then get yourself to the hairdressers and they will be able to cover up the part of your head that was shaved. Your finger can be put into a more comfortable splint in a couple of days, too. The fractured tailbone is going to cause you the most problem for a while, so it might be good to get away where you won't have the responsibilities of all your household chores.

continues

Case Study continued

Let someone else do all your cooking and cleaning. Traveling with a comfortable pillow to sit on is the only suggestion I might make to you."

"But what in the world will I do in the meantime? Look at all the dried blood still matted in my hair. This is awful."

"My assistant will be able to get a lot of that out for you. She can get most of it; the rest will have to wait until the stitches are removed. Then you can have it shampooed."

"What a relief that would be. Maybe we still can take a little trip. Maybe even our poodle will be well enough to be gone for a while, too. I'm certain I'll need some information from you for the dog-owner's insurance. Will I be able to get that?"

"You call me and I'll be glad to supply anything that is required. Let me know if you have any problems with your injuries. I see that you are scheduled for your annual physical soon. Let's set that appointment for the first part of next month so we can check everything again for you."

Mrs. Nelson left the clinic with her hair a little cleaner, reassurances from her physician, recognition of the trauma she had been through, and another appointment. The therapeutic relationship will continue.

STOP AND CONSIDER

Refer to Appendix A (see p. 224) and Maslow's Hierarchy of Needs.

Can you identify how and when the physician in this example elevated Mrs. Nelson's hierarchy of needs?

1.   In what level of need did the conversation begin?
2.   In what level of need did it end?
3.   How does Maslow's Hierarchy of Needs relate to those needs identified in Welter's levels of needs?

SUMMARY

The helping interview is a critical component of any therapeutic help-ing relationship. First impressions are very important, and last much longer than any care that is given to clients. Every action, every word, every experience is imprinted upon the participating client, who will experience either a positive or a negative reaction to the process. Health care professionals who perform this interview many times daily are to be constantly reminded that this is the first time for their client, and that their full attention is required. Giving full attention means that the health care professional sets aside any personal agenda to make certain that the client's needs are met and that necessary information is gained.

EXERCISES

Exercise 1

The following statement identifies personal appearance appropriate for health care professionals. Do you agree or disagree? Explain your rationale. Recall a negative and a positive experience with a health care professional that was reflected by that professional's personal appearance.

A daily bath, an effective deodorant, and fresh breath are essential personal characteristics. Hair that is clean, off the collar, and out of the face is both sanitary and easy to care for. Even the most attractive hair should not be on the collar while at work. Nails should be trimmed and neatly manicured. Any polish worn should be clear only. Hands must be washed between appointments with clients. Any uniform worn should fit properly and be appropriate for the setting. No aftershave or cologne should be worn. Men who are clean-shaven may be more acceptable to some clients than those with beards. It is best to wear no jewelry, with the exception of post earrings and wedding bands. Multiple body piercings and tattoos are offensive to many clients; therefore, they should be eliminated or kept covered whenever possible.

Exercise 2

Consider what your response might be to the following client statements made in the interview process.

1. "I want to have my sister come in with me for the examination."
    Response_____

2. "Yeah, those are my meds, but I stopped taking the little green ones because they upset my stomach."
    Response_____

3. "Why do I have to get on the scale every time I come here? It is embarrassing."
    Response_____

4. "You're not going to have to give little Johnnie a shot, are you?"
   Response_____

5. "Why won't you tell me the test results? Why do I have to wait for the doctor?"
   Response_____

6. "My best friend died of a heart attack this year. Can you do an EKG just to make sure everything is okay?"
   Response_____

7. "My wife made me come for this physical exam; otherwise, I wouldn't be here."
   Response_____

Exercise 3: Journal Exercise

1. Keep a journal every day for a week. In this journal, be aware of just one person who might have a problem. Can you identify the level of need? How about your own problems? Can you identify the levels of need and the helping responses?

2. Be aware of roadblocks to communication that you create or that you observe in other conversations. Make a note of these in your journal and identify how the roadblock could be changed to a helping response.

To be successful in these exercises, you will probably need to review daily the material in this unit that identifies levels of need and roadblocks.

Exercise 4

Identify the following as closed or open-ended questions, indirect statements, or roadblocks.

1. _____ How are you feeling today?

2. _____ You're looking pretty chipper today.

3. _____ Why did you do that?

4. _____ When I lift your leg, does it hurt?

5. _____ Oh, don't worry; everything will be fine.

6. _____ You're not getting old.

7. _____ Oh, it couldn't possibly feel like that.

8. _____ You say the accident happened this morning?

9. _____ What did the doctor tell you about the test results?

10. _____ Tell me about the test results.

11. _____ Could you tell me when you think this started?

12. _____ I'd like to hear about your new job.

13. _____ Why do you think you feel this way?

REVIEW QUESTIONS

Multiple Choice

1. The three components of the helping interview are

    a. greeting, identifying client's problem, and doctor's visit.

    b. orientation of each other, identifying the problem, and resolution of problem.

    c. open communication, hearing the problem, and clinic follow-up.

    d. orientation, open communication, and resolution of problem.

2. The orientation phase of the helping interview should find the health care professional using the following skills:

    a. sharing observations, acknowledging feelings, clarifying and validating, reflecting and paraphrasing.

    b. giving advice, requiring explanations, seeking approval, correcting, and defending.

    c. showing warmth, being genuine, establishing trust, and expressing sympathy/ empathy and sincerity.

    d. introducing client to the clinic, reviewing client's medical chart, discussing billing procedures, and monitoring insurance claims.

3. An indirect statement

    a. does not require the client to enlarge upon the response.

    b. can usually be answered with a *yes* or a *no.*

    c. encourages clients to identify more of the problem.

    d. calls for a client response without the client feeling questioned.

4. With today's changes in health care, it is important to

    a. empower the client to actively participate in his/ her health care.

    b. maintain the same health care provider through the adult years.

c. pay close attention to television ads for drugs and medicines.

d. have clients pay as much of their health care costs as possible.

5. When conducting the helping interview, it is best to

a. have the client sit on the examination table.

b. address the client informally to ease his/her anxiety.

c. not have the client disrobed during the interview orientation.

d. dress casually so the client is not intimidated.

FOR FURTHER CONSIDERATION

1. With another person in your class, identify ways in which the orientation phase of the helping interview with James Alonzo could be more productive and provide better care management. Once you have identified the changes you would make, role-play the orientation for your class.

2. What action might be taken to reduce James Alonzo's dislike of seeing a doctor and having a physical examination? How might the medical office assistant encourage him?

3. Gather as much information as you can about what medically oriented Web sites are most reputable and why. What questions would you ask yourself before relying upon a particular site? What kind of information can you share with clients who regularly use the Internet for information? Identify the particular sites you would recommend and justify your choices.

CASE STUDIES

Case Study 1

Alice Jameson is a 69-year-old who has been suffering with flu-like symptoms for several days. She calls her primary care provider to make an appointment. This conversation follows:

"Mid-Town Medical Clinic, this is Marianne; please hold." After a two- to three-minute wait, the receptionist comes back on the line.

"Thank you for holding. Can I help you?"

"This is Alice Jameson. I am feeling terrible. I think I have the flu. But I shouldn't have the flu; I got the flu shot last fall. Can I see my doctor?"

"Alice, we are so busy with flu patients, I don't have an opening until day after tomorrow. Can you come at 3:30 p.m.?"

After a brief pause, Alice responds, hesitantly.

> "No, I don't think so. If I don't get better, I guess I'll go to my neighborhood emergency care clinic."

> "Okay. Bye."

The receptionist at Mid-Town Medical Clinic does not learn that Alice has had a fever of 101 degrees for two days and does not recall that she had surgery to place an artificial heart valve just eight months ago.

Discuss this case study. Identify Alice's need. Were those needs met? Name the problems that exist in this situation. Then role-play a helping interview that can be therapeutic *and* can meet Alice's needs. Assume that the clinic's schedule really is full.

Case Study 2

At the close of a presurgical examination, it is your responsibility to bring the client written instructions related to hospital admission and presurgery preparations. As you present the information to Mia Trong, you sense that she may still have some questions. She seems hesitant to leave. What will you say? What will you do? What steps do you take to make certain Mia's questions have all been addressed?

RESOURCES

Desmond, J., & Copeland, L. R. (2000). *Communicating with today's patient*. San Francisco, CA: Jossey-Bass.

Libster, M. (2001). *Demonstrating care: the art of integrative nursing*. Albany, NY: Thomson Delmar Learning.

Schuster, P. M. (2000). *Communication: the key to the therapeutic relationship*. Philadelphia, PA: F. A. Davis Company.

Welter, P. (1990). *How to help a friend*. Wheaton, IL: Tyndale House Publishing.

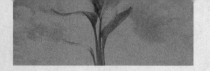

CHAPTER

4

THE THERAPEUTIC RESPONSE ACROSS THE LIFE SPAN

CHAPTER OBJECTIVES

The learner should strive to meet the following chapter objectives and demonstrate an understanding of the facts and principles presented in this chapter through written and oral communication.

- Define the key term as presented in the glossary.

- Compare/contrast Pavlov's theory with Skinner's theory. (Appendix A on p. 224)

- Describe Jean Piaget's theory of cognitive development. (Appendix A on p. 224)

- Discuss examples of the use of Piaget's theory of cognitive development in therapeutic communication. (Appendix A on p. 224)

- Describe Sigmund Freud's psychosocial forces—the id, the ego, and the superego. (Appendix A on p. 224)

- Describe Lawrence Kohlberg's moral development theory. (Appendix A on p. 224)

- Discuss appropriate methods health care professionals might use to encourage a healthy lifestyle as part of moral development.

- Discuss Erik Erikson's eight stages of psychosocial crises and appropriate therapeutic responses. (Appendix A on p. 224)

- Identify a minimum of five characteristics each that are particular to infants, children, adolescents, adults, and the elderly.
- Describe at least four guidelines for therapeutic communication for each age group, giving an example of how each might be instituted.
- Discuss the concept that, to be truly therapeutic, health care professionals must genuinely like their work and the age groups they are treating.

OPENING CASE STUDY

Dr. Charles Lewien, CEO of a large family practice clinic, was preparing a seminar for presentation to staff members on the subject of how to improve client communication. While musing on these thoughts, he was surprised by the circular nature of the life span encompassed by the clients seen at the clinic. Infants are totally dependent on caregivers and communicate by reactions to discomfort and pain and by touch. Children can vocalize but are very present focused, and often fearful. These behaviors require communication at a low level of understanding. Adolescents present a wall, separating them from all adults, and vary from behaving as a child one moment and as an adult the next. Adults would seem to be the easiest to communicate with, but they are frequently blindsided by their own concerns with raising a family, careers, and sexuality, making communication difficult. The elderly bring the communication problem full circle, as they become less independent, losing cognitive ability and experiencing decreasing mental sharpness. Dr. Lewien pondered whether any communication techniques are consistently applicable to each age group.

INTRODUCTION

The health care professional should have a sound background in and understanding of biological human growth and development, and must, of necessity, consider these principles when communicating with others.

To communicate therapeutically, helping professionals must consider a person's lifetime experiences, conditioning, predisposition and inherited characteristics, life cycle and span, relationship to others, learning abilities and vocation, and cultural background.

Many prominent theories of human growth and development and psychology exist. Of all the theories known, no *one* theory is generally accepted. Perhaps this is because, as Carl Rogers, the psychotherapist, believes, we are still in process. We are still learning and developing more viable and creative ways to live and work.

The goal of any health care professional must be to enable individuals to get in touch with themselves, to encourage them to discover a full and functioning life with meaning and purpose. Therefore, the more the health care professional knows and understands about human growth and development, the better prepared he/she will be to offer therapeutic communication. The opening case study concerning Dr. Lewien illustrates the progression of communication in the human life span.

❧ CASE STUDY ❧

John and Hannah Adams have had their first child, a son, home from the hospital just three days. John calls the pediatrician because he is worried about circumcision care. He noticed the formation of a yellow crust on the penis. Their son had a Gomco circumcision prior to leaving the hospital. The pediatrician reassures John that the crusted exudate is commonly seen on the glans penis and is normal and often observed during the healing process. The Adamses are encouraged to express any future concerns and to continue their good care of their son.

INFANTS

The preceding case study illustrates the therapeutic response to the infant caregiver: the medical professional explains the normal healing process, encourages the Adamses to continue the good care of their son and to feel free to call with any other health concerns. If the infant communicates discomfort by crying or being fussy, checking for signs of infection may be necessary. Infants are totally dependent upon their caregivers and have limited means of communicating their needs.

The infant stage of growth and development is very rapid and covers the time period from birth to 1 year of age. Physical comfort and safety are primary considerations during this phase of growth, since the infant cannot communicate his or her needs with spoken words. A therapeutic response to the infant consists of close observation and touch, which enhances the bonding process between the caregiver and infant and stimulates the infant.

THE THERAPEUTIC RESPONSE

Safety issues should be a primary concern. Infants can easily roll off tables and counters, so never take your eyes or hands off them. Observe what is within reach of infants, and prevent them grabbing or kicking items that could be a hazard.

Infants should be held lovingly for a few minutes on each visit, and especially after every painful procedure. They are sensitive to touch and need warmth and love. Holding them will help the infant associate the health care professional with feelings other than pain.

At about 3 months, infants begin to recognize familiar faces and voices. When possible, include the parent or caregiver in procedures, as security for the infant. Speaking in a soft, calm voice reassures the infant and caregiver.

Create an environment that is pleasant for the infant. At 8 months, the infant is developing a memory. Wearing colorful uniform tops or jackets or large buttons for interest helps create a pleasant atmosphere. Mobiles hung appropriately in the examination room add interest and may divert the infant's attention to something pleasurable.

Be aware of family characteristics and history. Medical professionals will find it helpful to have an understanding of the ethnic, cultural, and family background of the infant. This information assists in interpreting apparent irregularities in the infant's growth and development. For example, Asian infants typically have a lower birth weight and are shorter than the lengths given on normal development charts, which are biased toward the majority European American population. In similar fashion, Native American infants are frequently heavier at birth than European American infants. Genetic patterns present in one or both parents can be critical to understanding developmental problems. Medical professionals must be aware of these factors to provide the necessary therapeutic response beneficial to both the infant and the caregiver.

Parents and caregivers often have questions about infant care. Take the time to listen carefully to their questions and concerns. Restate the question or concern to validate and clarify that you have heard correctly. Respond to each question or concern by providing information, instructing, or demonstrating procedures to educate the parent or caregiver.

STOP AND CONSIDER

Reread the infant case study and respond to the following questions.

1. What questions might be asked to assess the infant's health status?
2. How was the pediatrician therapeutic in response to John's concerns?
3. How does the case study reflect B.F. Skinner's theory of operant conditioning?

❧ CASE STUDY ❧

Katie is going to the doctor today. She is 2½ years old. She is excited about going because they have such great toys for her. When she arrives with her grandma, she goes straight for the toys. The wait is not long; when the medical assistant is ready, she calls Katie by name. In the examination room, the physician talks directly to Katie, and allows her to play with the stethoscope and to listen to her heartbeat. Katie is not afraid and likes the physician.

CHILDREN

Any person may have difficulty adjusting to being ill and to being under the care of a physician. Children may have an even more difficult time, because they do not fully understand what is happening to them. Children cannot comprehend why the medicine or treatment is going to help them feel better. Some children even feel they are being punished or have done something terribly wrong when they are ill.

Children, like all human beings, fear what they do not know or understand. Even the smallest procedure seems major. Parents, adults, and health care professionals who take the time to explain what is happening and to increase a child's knowledge are apt to have a soothing effect and reduce their anxiety. Having a consistent routine during visits allows the child to anticipate what to expect, and reduces their fear.

A health care professional should consider the relationship between children and the parents or primary caregivers. A good relationship with caregivers will lessen the problems with their children.

THE THERAPEUTIC RESPONSE

The environment is important for children. Pediatric offices should be colorful, attractive, and comfortable. There should be safe and clean toys to keep their minds active and distracted from procedures.

The health care professional should establish a friendly relationship with each child. This is accomplished by focusing attention on the child. Kneel in front of children, make eye contact, and speak directly to them on their level of understanding. Mention something positive about the shirt or shoes they are wearing or ask something about the teddy bear they are holding. A positive approach, praise for accomplishments, and acknowledgment of desirable behaviors is much more effective than negative or critical approaches.

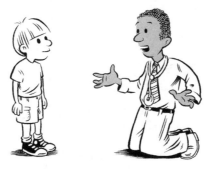

"WOW! LET ME LOOK AT THOSE NEW TENNIS SHOES."

Give a child a choice only when you know the decision will be the correct one. For example, "Shall we see how tall you are first or how much you weigh?" It makes no difference which choice is made; both procedures will be accomplished. Let children help with procedures if you can, but do not lose control of the situation. Johnny may hold the tape while you apply the bandage to his leg.

Do not keep children and their parents waiting. They become anxious quickly. Visits to the doctor's office that are short, have some pleasant experiences, and have friendly, caring health care professionals whom children recognize are the most effective visits.

Help children deal with their feelings. When children ask questions, respond in short, simple answers. Be truthful and honest. Children who become angry and frustrated can hit a doll, pound clay, or draw pictures. Do not expect to be rewarded by children for the examination, especially if it involves anything painful. In fact, children may tell you they do not like you.

Listen to the feelings children express, verbally or nonverbally. Learn as much about pediatric clients as possible from parents. Recognize that crying and silence are pleas for comfort and care as well as anger and frustration.

continues

The Therapeutic Response continued

Listen to parents' concerns. Respond truthfully, even if the facts may be upsetting. Help parents deal with their children's feelings and behavior. Encourage them to reinforce with warmth and tenderness rather than fear and anxiety.

Give rewards. They can be simple; a hug, even a hand-shake or high-five is good. Children especially enjoy balloons, stickers, and hand stamps. One pediatric office is known by children as the office of "stamps"—they have over fifty to choose from. At the end of each visit, a child selects two: one to be stamped on each hand.

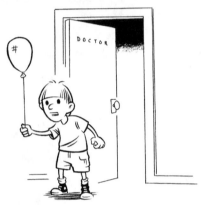

"LOOK WHAT I GOT!"

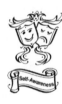

Be aware of your own feelings when approaching children. They know instantly if you are insecure or do not like them. Children can be "unlovable" when they are frustrated, angry, and in pain. You must be personally able to handle their feelings.

Working with children is a challenge, but one that, fortunately, many dedicated health care professionals enjoy. Keep in mind these guidelines and remember to always enjoy your profession.

STOP AND CONSIDER

1. Identify therapeutic responses or actions the medical assistant and the physician incorporated to help Katie feel more comfortable during her visit today.
2. Consult Appendix A on p. 224 to determine which of Piaget's cognitive development learning theories Katie is currently experiencing.
3. Why is it important to develop a consistent routine during office visits for this age group?

CASE STUDY

Taking Jeff, age 14, to the pediatrician as a teenager was different from when he was younger. As they were driving there, Jeff's mom asked if he would prefer to see the doctor alone. Jeff's immediate response was "Yes." His mom assured him that she was there if he needed her. When they arrived, Jeff quickly picked up one of the car magazines that the office staff had available and promptly ignored the two children playing in the child's corner.

When Jeff was called, he proudly marched to the examination room alone. During the examination, the physician posed a question that he always asked of teenagers: "Jeff, are you sexually active?" Jeff, a little embarrassed, responded negatively, but the physician hastened to go on. "It is a question I ask all my teenage clients, and I'll ask you when you are in next year. It is important for me to have a truthful answer. It is good you are not yet sexually active. Girls are wonderful; sex is wonderful; but both are addicting." Jeff laughed. The ice had been broken for future discussions regarding sex.

ADOLESCENTS

Adolescence is a period of transition from childhood to adulthood. Adolescents fight for their independence, yet have the same needs for comfort and security as children. It is a turbulent time for teenagers, as well as for their parents and primary caregivers.

Many demands are placed on adolescents. The demands come from family, school, peers, and society. The bodies of adolescents are changing. They are awkward and feel unsure of themselves. They are confused by their sexual feelings. It is a time when it is vitally important that the adolescent have something to feel good about.

The problems adolescents face often seem insurmountable to them. They may suffer from unsightly acne. Many girls have painful menstruation. Boys may begin to have nocturnal emissions. There is an enormous amount of pressure from peers, who often have a misguided notion or fantasy of what an adolescent is expected to be.

Another reason this is a difficult period is that parents, who are often occupied with earning a living and making a career for themselves while supporting their families, are also perplexed with the sudden changes in their adolescent sons and daughters. Teenagers and their parents are likely to have opposing views on just about everything.

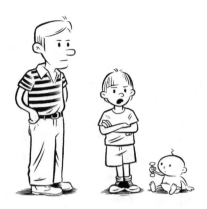

"WHY CAN'T I DRIVE?"

THE THERAPEUTIC RESPONSE

Allow the adolescent privacy and the right to be examined or treated without parents present. It is best not to moralize, but to generate an atmosphere in which the teenager will feel comfortable enough to ask questions and seek information.

Do not assume that parents have told their teenagers everything they need to know about sex. Use correct anatomical and socially accepted terms for genitalia and sexual expressions, and provide accurate and factual information through books, pamphlets, and videos. Not only do adolescents need to understand their sexuality physiologically and emotionally, they also must understand safe sex and the responsibility that goes with being sexually active. Health care professionals often avoid this topic, but events in today's society no longer allow such an attitude.

Treat adolescents with respect and dignity. Ask open-ended questions about their worries and concerns and avoid making comments about their clothes or hairstyle or speaking about good grades as the only important endeavor. Find out what is important in their lives, how they like to spend their time, and what kind of concerns they have. Make notes on their chart so you can bring up the topic at their next visit.

Set limits that are fair and consistent. Discourage antisocial behavior while encouraging self-control and establishment of identity. Do not take sides in a teenager's battle with parents. Help both parent and teenager assess and understand their positions.

You must clearly like and care about adolescents. If you do not, you will be ineffective in being therapeutic. You cannot hide your feelings from children and adolescents.

Set the stage for the adolescent's transfer from pediatric care to adult care. Young adults often struggle in this transition to establish a relationship with a personal physician. During college years or their first years of employment, young adults are often away from home and have only minimal financial resources. Help instill in their minds the importance of quality health care throughout their lifetime.

continues

The Therapeutic Response continued

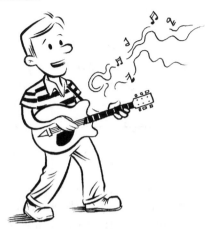

**"HOW COME YOU'RE ALWAYS
TELLING ME WHAT TO DO."**

Adolescents need to feel a sense of worth. They need time and understanding to resolve the tensions they feel. The health care professional can be a positive force in this direction. Adolescents welcome established limits that offer security but allow them to gain a little bit of adulthood. Listen to the adolescent; you may be surprised at what you learn.

STOP AND CONSIDER

Recall the case study about Jeff's visit to the doctor's office.

1. How might it be different to take Jeff to the doctor as a child compared to as an adolescent?
2. Review Freud's psychosexual stages of development as presented in Appendix A on p. 224. Freud theorized that each individual's behavior consists of three major forces: the id, the ego, and the superego. Which force do you think is more prominent in Jeff's life as an adolescent?

❧ CASE STUDY ❧

Karen, a 40-year-old mother, presents for her annual physical examination. As the assistant is recording Karen's vital signs and taking a chief complaint, she asks how everything else is going. Karen relates some difficulty dealing with a teenage daughter who is not doing well in school and whose

continues

Case Study continued

behavior is troublesome. The assistant responds, "That is quite a worry, isn't it? Your doctor has a lot of skills in helping parents cope with teenagers. Let me mention your concern to him. Also, we have some wonderful pamphlets at the front desk that might help. I'll collect some for you to take home."

Karen is relieved that she will be able to talk with someone about her concerns. She is feeling like such a failure as a parent right now.

ADULTS

Many of the principles applied to children and adolescents are appropriate for adults of all ages. Adults should be recognized for the characteristic activities of this age group—working toward life's vocation, earning a living, establishing primary relationships, making a place for themselves in a community, and perhaps raising a family.

Because these activities require an inordinate amount of responsibility, a fair amount of stress-related complaints will be found in this age group. This group can also benefit from information and assistance regarding daily living and parenting. For instance, if a child suffers from a chronic illness, the astute and therapeutic physician recognizes the need to also care for the parents. Education will be an important component of each helping interview.

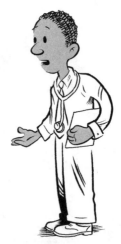

"THE LAB WAS CONCERNED
ONE OF YOUR LAB VALUES
WAS LOW."

Younger adults may actually be living in an extended psychological adolescent period, since many are still pursuing an education or are not independent from parents. However, the fact that these young adults are physically mature and are most likely living an adult life in all other ways is a source of conflict to be recognized.

Physically, persons in this age group are quite healthy. Women are apt to be bearing children in the younger adult years or facing menopause in their 40s and 50s. Men will pass through a period identified as climacteric, when their hormone production tends to slow and diminish.

It is especially crucial during the adult years to recognize the unequal partnership occurring between client and physician and to equalize the relationship as much as possible. Therefore, keep the following recommendations in mind.

THE THERAPEUTIC RESPONSE

Get to know adult clients. Never allow a therapeutic interview to pass without a discussion of what is happening in the client's life. As much care will be given with an honest discussion of daily occurrences as from a discussion of a particular ailment or chief complaint.

Recognize the skills and intelligence of clients and do not try to impress them by unnecessary use of medical nomenclature. Explain in terms clients will understand and comprehend. Do not, in any way, talk down to clients. Recognize the client's desire for information and knowledge regarding treatment and care.

Emphasize preventive health care. While most adults see the physician for a "cure" or treatment for an ailment, use that opportunity to educate clients regarding preventive health measures. This is the life stage when prevention can save time and money and lead to better health in the later adult years.

Recognize your role as a member of the health care team. Adults are likely to have more than one primary care physician. Consider the woman who receives care during pregnancy and delivery from an OB/GYN and staff, but still sees a family physician for all other care. This duplication should complement rather than conflict.

Recognize the stress caused by any accident or serious illness in this age group. This is the age identified as the "prime of life." Any serious ailment or accident is apt to be met with anger, **denial**, and depression. People in this age group do not think about death or disability; they put off such thoughts for the later adult years.

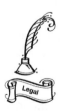

Respect clients' right to privacy. Clients have a right to expect that the information shared with health care professionals is protected. Adults often reveal information that could compromise their reputation if known to others. Confidentiality must always be preserved.

Encourage adult clients to hope for the best, but do not promise specific results. Health care professionals cannot predict a sure outcome and should never do so. Promising a cure only destroys the therapeutic relationship if or when the cure does not occur.

STOP AND CONSIDER

Review the adult case study, then respond to the following questions.

1. Which of Erikson's psychosocial stages of development is Karen in at the present time?
2. Do you think the assistant responded appropriately to Karen's comments about her daughter? Justify your answer.

CASE STUDY

Mr. Levine is 78 years of age. He has just learned that he has prostate cancer and must have radiation treatment. He is confused about what all this means. Using an anatomical picture, the physician shows Mr. Levine where the cancer is located. He tells him that the good news is that the examination showed the cancer was not advanced, nor had it spread.

Carefully, treatment is detailed. Mr. Levine asks the physician to write some of this down so he will be able to tell his daughter what is happening. The physician complies and tells him what to expect from the treatment. Mr. Levine leaves the office with an appointment to see the radiologist, but not until the assistant has told him to feel free to call any time with any questions he might have.

ELDER ADULTS

Older adults experience fewer acute illnesses. However, chronic illnesses, such as hypertension, diabetes, arthritis, and hearing and vision impairment, often plague this age group. At the same time, a loss of self-identity and feelings of belonging often occur when a person retires and/or experiences lifestyle changes.

The elderly may look forward to this period as a time of more freedom, a time to pursue activities they never accomplished in their younger years, and a time of fewer obligations. Others may look at this final stage as a time when they no longer feel needed, a time when they become bored and lack the energy to participate in new activities, and a time of fear for the loss of personal safety, financial security, and good health.

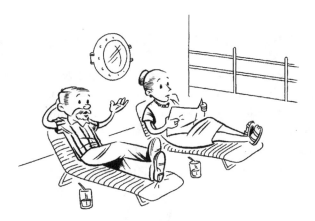

**"I'M GLAD I RETIRED.
THIS IS THE LIFE."**

The way younger years have been spent is likely the same way the later years will be spent. If a person has been active and involved, has been a member of one or more organizations, and has had many friends, the same activities usually continue. The individual who preferred to be alone, had few interests, and was not a member of any organization generally prefers the same lifestyle in later years. Some, especially those in business for themselves, find retirement difficult if they have no hobbies or interests. Illness, loss of a loved one, or relocation can disrupt this pattern and result in depression or withdrawal.

All of the guidelines mentioned for a therapeutic response for the adult population should be carried through for the elderly as well. Some additional guidelines are appropriate.

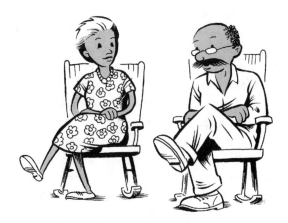

**"TOO BAD WE DON'T HAVE MONEY
FOR THAT CRUISE. GUESS WE'LL
HAVE TO ROCK AND DREAM."**

THE THERAPEUTIC RESPONSE

Allow additional time for the elderly to compensate for physiological changes. This client requires more time to ambulate or to disrobe or dress, and may need assistance. More care should be taken in explaining procedures. Talk slowly and clearly. Allow for any sensory deprivation and do not be afraid to raise questions regarding a sensory loss to assess how a client might be better treated. Some are too embarrassed to ask about a hearing loss, for instance, but are relieved when a physician discusses it.

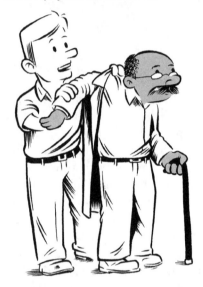

"LET ME HELP YOU WITH YOUR COAT."

Comfort is important at this age. Be sure the reception room furniture is comfortable. It is easier for older people to rise from a firm, straight-backed chair with arms than from a soft, low sofa. Assess whether the examination rooms are adaptable to the elderly. Provide pillows for support and comfort. Handrails in the restroom provide security and support and allow the elderly freedom to be autonomous.

A set schedule is often best. The elderly are comfortable and secure in a routine. Allow for that routine. If a person must be seen weekly to monitor blood pressure, ask that he/she come in on the same day at the same time each week.

Elderly persons are to be treated with respect and with the recognition that their lives are valuable. Do not operate under the assumption that "since you've lived a full life, you probably won't want to..." Treatment is as important to the elderly as it is to youth.

Do not be oversolicitous or overprotective. This only serves to reduce self-esteem and intensify the feelings the elderly may be having. Verbal and nonverbal communication can help the client retain self-esteem and confidence during the elder years. Ask what the clients like and dislike about the office and care.

continues

The Therapeutic Response continued

Interest elderly clients in activities as much as possible. A discussion of their daily activities helps to assess if they might benefit from additional activity in their lives. In making suggestions, consider their aptitude, physical abilities, and interests. Be aware of appropriate referrals, such as adult day care, senior citizens' centers, etc.

Help the elderly client remain independent as long as possible. However, do not be afraid to honestly indicate when it is time for additional care or altered living situations. Talking with clients to determine what kind of plans they have for the time when they can no longer adequately care for themselves is beneficial in helping clients make their own decisions.

Remember the needs of the primary caregivers of the elderly. Whether caring for the elderly in an "at-home" environment or in one of the many institutional facilities available today, the primary caregivers must have a respite. A weekend or even a day free of caregiving responsibility is revitalizing and necessary for all parties concerned.

Understand your own feelings toward aging parents or growing older yourself. Try to determine how you would like to be treated and provide the same courtesy to your older clients. The entire staff has the responsibility of helping the elderly feel needed and wanted.

Remember that some diseases/disorders may affect cognition. Cognition refers to processes by which a person knows the world and interacts with it. Cognition involves the way in which the brain learns and interprets information. The human brain is a very delicate and sensitive organ that is susceptible to injury from both internal and external factors, such as falls causing blows to the head, which may result in brain injury. The use and/or side effects of some drugs, electrolyte imbalance, and ischemia caused by some disease processes are examples of external factors affecting brain function. Therapeutic responses must allow for the cognitive aspect.

STOP AND CONSIDER

1. Identify therapeutic responses or actions the physician incorporated to help Mr. Levine understand his health care problem and treatment plan.
2. Consult Appendix A on p. 224 to determine which of Erikson's eight psychosocial crises Mr. Levine is progressing through.
3. What other therapeutic responses and/or actions are important to remember when working with this age group?

SUMMARY

Understanding human growth and development is essential for health care professionals if they are to communicate effectively with their clients. Lifetime experiences, education, predisposition and inherited characteristics, and culture are also important factors to be considered. The more the health care professional knows and understands about growth and development, the better prepared he/she will be to offer therapeutic responses. Therapeutic communication should be aimed toward helping clients get in touch with themselves and encouraging them to discover a full and functioning life with meaning and purpose.

One of the concepts identified throughout the various age groups is the idea that, to be effective in therapeutic communication, health care professionals must genuinely like their work and the age groups they are treating. That concept might be applied to any vocation that requires contact with the public as its base. However, dealing with persons who are ill, in pain, or may be dying is quite different than the professional who is making your travel arrangements to go to Paris for a vacation.

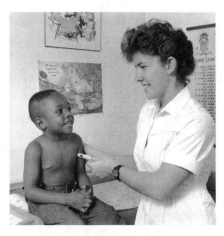
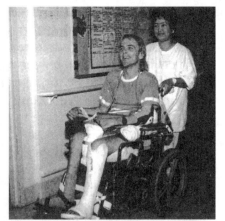
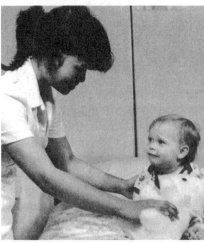
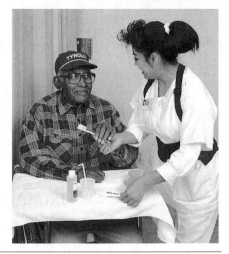

FIGURE 4-1 Accept each client in accordance with his or her stage of development.

Because health care is such serious business, it is even more important for professionals to like their work. Having a healthy respect for life and for each age group and its particular problems, and a mature notion regarding dying and death is a must for effective therapeutic communications. See Figure 4-1.

EXERCISES

Exercise 1

In groups of three, identify your personal worst experience in a health care setting. Role-play with a group member how that situation could be turned from your worst experience into one that was therapeutic. Have the third person judge the therapeutic response.

Continue role-playing until each of you has shared a worst experience and identified how to make it therapeutic.

Exercise 2

Interview an elderly person, an adolescent, and an adult. Ask the following questions:

1. When you last visited your physician, how were you treated?

2. What did you like the best?

3. What did you dislike?

4. Why do you seek care from this particular physician?

Exercise 3

Visit a pediatric, children's, or hospice wing in a local hospital. Observe the patients' needs and the therapeutic responses offered to these patients by the professionals and paraprofessionals who care for them. Write a brief summary expressing your comfort level with the age group and outlining the therapeutic responses you might have offered in that situation.

Exercise 4

Search the Internet for information about one or more of the age groups discussed in this chapter. Print out or prepare a list of

- telephone numbers and addresses that you might contact for literature.

- Internet sites, books, videos, or other media that age groups discussed in this chapter might be interested in researching.

- resources for families needing support information for these age groups.

- government Web sites for information on seniors' health care, Medicaid, Medicare, and support groups.

REVIEW QUESTIONS

Multiple Choice

1. Piaget's theory was termed

   a. Cognitive Development.

   b. Psychosexual Stages of Development.

   c. Humanistic Psychology.

   d. Psychosocial Crises.

2. Sigmund Freud's id is also known as

   a. the ego.

   b. the superego.

   c. the pleasure principle.

   d. the reality principle.

3. All of the following are true about erogenous zones *except* that

   a. they include the mouth, anus, and genital organs.

   b. they are regions of the body more likely to experience tensions that can be relieved by action upon the region.

   c. they are associated with the satisfaction of a vital need.

   d. they are considered of little importance for personality development.

4. Pediatric health care offices should keep all of the following in mind *except* that

   a. they should be colorful, attractive, and comfortable.

   b. they should have a variety of magazines for children to read.

   c. they should have safe, clean toys for children to play with.

   d. professionals should use a positive approach, praise for accomplishments, and acknowledge desirable behaviors.

5. Which statement is false regarding adolescents?

   a. Adolescents fight for their independence, yet have the same needs for comfort and security as children.

   b. Health care professionals have a great influence on adolescents' moral development.

c. Health care professionals are often called upon to discuss a healthy lifestyle for teens.

d. Adolescents should be treated with respect and dignity.

6. Which statement is false regarding adults?

a. Many of the principles applied to children and adolescents are appropriate for adults of all ages.

b. Emphasize preventive health care with adults.

c. Privacy is not an issue to be considered with adults.

d. Explain illness and disease in terms the client will understand and comprehend.

7. All of the following are true of the elderly *except* that

a. they cannot live independently and are considered senile.

b. the elder years often reflect the lifestyle of younger years.

c. additional time should be allowed for the elderly to compensate for physiological changes.

d. A set schedule is best for the elderly.

FOR FURTHER CONSIDERATION

1. How can the health care professional prepare for working with various age groups?

2. Safety is an important issue for all age groups. How can you make your office safer for the various clients and visitors who frequent your facility?

3. How relevant is Freud's theory in today's health care setting?

4. Why is self-awareness such an important issue when working with the various age groups?

CASE STUDIES

Case Study 1

Catherine is 17½ years old. She has been seen by a pediatrician for childhood illnesses and checkups since she was born. Her mother and her grandmother have both had thyroid cancer; since this a familial disorder, there is concern for Catherine. Her mother has annual follow-ups with an endocrinologist and has asked Catherine if she would allow him to check her blood and do an examination. This information could then be sent to the new internal medicine physician Catherine will be seeing as an adult.

1. How might her mother engage in conversation with Catherine? She does not want to cause undue concern or frighten Catherine.

2. Assuming Catherine agrees to visit the endocrinologist, how might he approach Catherine therapeutically?

3. What are some important considerations to think about when working with teenagers?

Case Study 2

Jim has a family history of coronary artery disease. His father had a massive heart attack and died at age 38. His twin brother had quadruple bypass surgery at age 42, and Jim had a mild heart attack at age 46. He has changed his lifestyle to reduce stress and include daily exercise; eats healthy, well-balanced meals; and monitors his cholesterol levels regularly. For the past three months, however, Jim has been experiencing atrial fibrillation and arrhythmia.

An important business meeting had Jim hurrying out the door with no time for breakfast and with a 50-minute drive into the city through gridlock traffic. It was past lunchtime when he headed for home. While driving, he felt dizzy and pulled to the side of the freeway. He realized his heart was not functioning properly, but he had no chest pain or nausea. He called his cardiologist and was told to call 911 or get to the ER immediately. Jim, in denial, drove himself to the hospital, since he was only a few minutes away.

As Jim crossed the lobby of the ER, he experienced another dizzy spell and crashed onto the counter. The receptionist asked him if that was his car in front of the door. He said, "Yes." The receptionist said, "You will have to move your car; you can't leave it there." Jim replied, "I'm having a heart attack, I need help!"

A passing nurse heard the comment and immediately went into action. Jim was soon on a gurney with six staff simultaneously poking and prodding his upper body.

An angiogram revealed that Jim had a 99 percent blockage in four of the main arteries of his heart, making quadruple bypass surgery a necessity. Jim is recovering nicely today and continues his healthy lifestyle.

1. How might the cardiologist have responded more therapeutically?

2. Was the receptionist's response appropriate?

3. How might the receptionist have been more therapeutic?

RESOURCES

Frisch, N. C., & Frisch, L. E. (2006). *Psychiatric mental health nursing*. Albany, NY: Thomson Delmar Learning.

Kalman, N., & Waughfield, C. G. (1998). *Mental health concepts* (4th ed.). Albany, NY: Thomson Delmar Learning.

Mandleco, B. L. (2004). *Growth & development handbook: newborn through adolescent*. Albany, NY: Thomson Delmar Learning.

Milliken, M. E., & Honeycutt, A. (2004). *Understanding human behavior: a guide for health care providers* (7th ed.). Albany, NY: Thomson Delmar Learning.

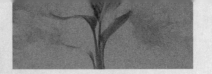

CHAPTER

5

THE THERAPEUTIC RESPONSE TO STRESSED AND ANXIOUS CLIENTS

CHAPTER OBJECTIVES

The learner should strive to meet the following chapter objectives and demonstrate an understanding of the facts and principles presented in this chapter through written and oral communication.

- Define the key terms as presented in the glossary.

- Differentiate between the terms *stress* and *stressor(s)*.

- Describe stress theories as presented by

  - Claude Bernard

  - Walter B. Cannon

  - Hans Selye

- Describe the impact of the stress response on the body.

- Identify the four levels of anxiety and describe each one.

- Identify signs and symptoms of normal and dysfunctional stress in each age group and list ways to decrease stress for each.

- Identify three therapeutic responses to normal stress and three therapeutic responses to dysfunctional stress for each age group.

- List a minimum of six ways to generally decrease stress.

John and Janice live in a small community and completed a first-aid class several weeks ago. As Janice washed the lunch dishes, she suddenly felt a sense of concern for the safety of her 5-year-old son, David, who was playing in the backyard. Hearing a scream, she ran to the window to see what had happened. Janice felt her heart pounding and her stomach became tied in knots. From the window, she saw David lying on the ground, motionless. He had fallen from the tree house where he often played.

When Janice reached David's side, she noticed how pale he was and that his voice was just a whimper. He felt cold and clammy, so she quickly removed her sweater and placed it gently around his limp body. Janice called to a neighbor to notify 911, and to bring some water and a washcloth. Janice comforted David and instructed him to lie still. When he asked for water, she gently touched his lips with the wet washcloth and then placed it on his forehead. David panted for air while Janice continued to speak softly to him and gently smoothed his hair back with her fingertips.

At the emergency room, X-rays revealed a broken leg, which was set and placed in a cast. David spent the night at the hospital for further observation, and was discharged the next day.

INTRODUCTION

The Chinese word for *crisis* is written by combining two symbols—one symbol meaning danger and the other meaning opportunity. Stress is just that: a danger and an opportunity, a friend and a foe. The term **stress** has been described as a nonspecific body response to a stressor. The stressor in the opening case study was the accident involving Janet's son, David.

STRESSORS AND STRESS

Stressors are internal perceptions or external events that cause the body's **autonomic nervous system** to respond, to protect the body. This places the body in a state of stress that can be beneficial or harmful, depending on severity and duration.

Internal stressors are products of emotions, and are referred to as anxieties. Internal stressors can be totally imaginary, having no relationship to real events. Memories (delayed stress syndrome) or nonthreatening real events can also trigger internal stressors. Internal stressors or anxieties cause a stress reaction in the body that is the same as that caused by external stressors. When these stressors are of long duration or severity, they become medically significant forms of mental illness. (See anxiety section on p. 115.)

External stressors result from external events or observations and involve a sensation of fright or fearfulness. The body's response is the same as for internal stressors, except that the duration of the stress is controlled by the external event. Most external stressors are of short duration. An example of a short-term external stressor would be a dog suddenly lunging toward you. An example of a long-term external stressor would be a soldier in continuous combat lasting days, weeks, or months. Initially the fear factor is very high, resulting in many soldiers "freezing" and experiencing an inability to react. With time, the external stressor becomes the norm.

Understanding the cause of stress is essential in order for stress management to be effective. The most common cause of stress is change; examples include relocation, loneliness, job loss, job promotion, retirement, divorce, bereavement, and illness. Health care professionals must understand the physical and mental trauma experienced by clients who are stressed and become ill. Improvements in medical technology and advances in health care may allow clients to experience a longer life expectancy even while suffering illness and disease. For some clients, an adjustment to the fact that they will never fully recover must be faced. They may also be forced to make decisions regarding lifestyle changes. For example: How long can they live independently? What financial security issues must be considered?

It is also important to remember the impact of stress's intensity and duration. The stress may be brief, as one would experience when temporarily misplacing the car keys. Cumulative stress may become chronic, depending on the intensity and duration of the stressor. For instance, some people live with chronic stress when caring for an elderly parent with Alzheimer's 24-7, or when enduring an abusive relationship that seems inescapable.

It is interesting to note that men and women respond differently to stress. Men often become physically or verbally aggressive, and may also use denial as a defense mechanism. (See Appendix B.) Women, on the other hand, often internalize their stress, mulling it over and over again in their minds. This reaction may lead to depression if satisfactory solutions to the stress are not achieved. Children may express stress based on their stage of growth and development, or may reflect patterns of dealing with stress demonstrated by other family members or caregivers. Examples include shouting, throwing things, or behavior that acts out their frustration.

Most think of stress as being something bad or negative and unhealthy. Stress is a normal part of life; it is a useful response that may be termed **eustress** and is considered positive. We all need a certain amount of stress to remain alive and functioning at peak performance. Too much stress, however, is an enemy, and causes the body to malfunction.

STRESS THEORIES

Claude Bernard was a 19th-century French biologist who discovered that the body's **internal milieu** (internal environment) changed constantly to meet the daily demands of life. Blood pressure, heart rate, respiration, and the amount of available energy in the circulating blood supply fluctuate to maintain homeostasis. He also learned that if any of these changed too much, the body could not adapt, and death followed.

Sometimes outside agents, such as pathogens, injury and trauma, or environmental pollutants and contaminants, cause these changes to the body. Our bodies also have vulnerable spots. Disease and old injuries may leave weak areas that feel the impact of stress. The aging process in general makes us more susceptible to stress symptoms.

A Harvard physiologist, Walter B. Cannon, went a step further than Bernard. Cannon discovered that the body adjusts when change threatens to be too great. For example, when blood is lost through any means, the body compensates for the loss by causing small changes in blood vessels all over the body. The heart rate increases slightly and fluid is transferred from tissues to the bloodstream, to bring balance and homeostasis.

Cannon also discovered that when life-threatening situations arise, excitatory substances such as adrenaline, cholestrol, and glucose are released into the bloodstream. These adjustments cause the body to adapt, and greatly enhance the body's chances of survival. These substances prepare the body for effort and protect it from harm.

It was Hans Selye who first conceived the theory of nonspecific reactions as stress; he named his theory **General Adaptation Syndrome (GAS)**. Selye theorized that the body experiences three stages in its response to stress: 1) the reaction stage, 2) the adaptation stage, and 3) the exhaustion stage. If the body successfully endures the stress encounter, the **parasympathetic nervous system** is activated and the body slowly returns to normal.

The reaction stage is composed of an alarm response and a fight-or-flight response. The adaptation stage takes place if stress continues for an extended length of time. During this stage, body changes may take place to reduce the effect of the stressor: a starving person has less desire for food; soldiers in extended combat are less fearful of the death and destruction all around them. The adaptation stage cannot continue indefinitely without harm to the body. During the exhaustion stage, the body's resistance to the stressor diminishes and may completely fail, resulting in serious illness or death.

Selye also defined a resource he called **adaptive energy**. This energy influences the body's resistance to stress. It is inherited and varies from one individual to another. It consists of a superficial level that can be replenished at the conclusion of a stressful event and a deep level that is not replenished and, when depleted, results in disease or death.

The following paragraphs detail the four body responses Selye identified as part of GAS in Figure 5-1.

Alarm

The alarm stage is designed to sound a warning when something is perceived to create stress. Pain is a part of this system, as it tells us when body tissue is being damaged.

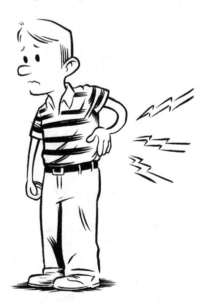

"OUCH!"

A therapeutic response in the medical office would be to recognize the fact that pain does produce a stress response. Ask the client to describe the pain and how it feels. Where is the pain located? Is the pain constant or intermittent? Offer suggestions for coping with pain. Often, breathing in through the nose and exhaling through the mouth will help. If the pain is caused by a procedure in progress, you may be able to distract and engage the client in conversation, or reassure the client that it will soon be finished.

Fight or Flight

The **sympathetic nervous system** prepares the body for fight or flight. The pupils dilate; the mouth becomes dry; the heart rate, pulse, and respiration all increase. Blood vessels in the skin constrict and blood vessels in the heart and brain dilate. There is decreased motility in the gastrointestinal and genitourinary tracts. All these changes prepare the body for whatever action may need to be taken.

Health care professionals should be alert for these signs and take all possible measures to decrease the stress response. Recognize that a certain amount of stress will be present no matter why the person is seeing the physician. Clients may be concerned about how a procedure or illness will affect their physical, mental, and emotional well-being. They may be frustrated or angry because they do not have a solution to a particular problem. As a health care professional, it is important not to take anger that may be directed at you personally. It should be treated as a sign and symptom of a client's stress. Provide privacy for those who may be asked to disrobe for an examination. Knock on the door before entering. Keep equipment, instruments, and syringes covered or out of sight. It is very stressful to come into an examination room, see such items, and wonder how they will be used.

Exhaustion

The body can only stay in the fight-or-flight state for a limited time. Have you ever stretched a rubber band to the maximum and held it there? After a while, your body tires of holding the stretched rubber band and releases it. When it is released, the band has lost some of its elasticity, which can never be recovered. The same principle applies to the blood vessels throughout the body. After repeated periods of dilation and relaxation, they are weakened. Also, if it is overstretched, the rubber band may snap. Blood vessels burst when they are dilated to an extreme or have developed weakened areas.

Individuals in this stage of stress may experience physical fatigue. It is best not to give detailed instructions at this time. Rather, allow them to recover—perhaps have them dress after the procedure and relax for a short while. If instructions must be given, it is best to write them out.

Return to Normal

During the return-to-normal stage, the parasympathetic nervous system kicks in and the body returns to normal. The pupils constrict; salivary glands begin to function; heart rate, pulse, and respiration decrease. Blood vessels dilate in the skin and constrict in the heart and brain. The gastrointestinal and genitourinary tracts begin to function again, and diarrhea may be experienced.

In the medical setting, these individuals respond well to a calm, soft voice. Encourage them to talk about how they are feeling and what helps them cope with the stress. Eye contact and active listening skills will help as well.

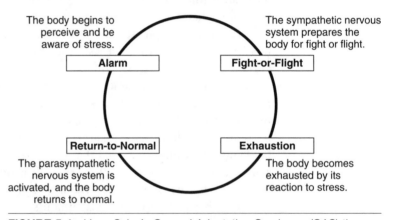

FIGURE 5-1 Hans Selye's General Adaptation Syndrome (GAS) theory proposes that four stages are involved in adapting to stress.

STRESS AND THE LIFE SPAN

We do not often stop to realize that infants experience stressors, just as much as older individuals. Early experiences greatly influence behavior patterns in later life. It is not so much what happens during infancy, but what does *not* happen that has an impact on behavioral patterns. An infant is totally dependent upon adults for survival. For the infant, the method of expressing stress is to cry. If the stress is not reduced and needs are not met, the only coping mechanism available to the infant is sleep.

To reduce stress, the infant's physical needs must be met. Health care professionals must recognize the fact that not all parents understand or have the basic skills and financial resources to meet these needs.

Providing resource information to parents and/or taking some time to teach and instruct is helpful and is more apt to ensure that the infant's needs are met. When parents fail to show interest in the infant and its needs are not satisfied, certain behavioral patterns are recognizable in the toddler stage. Often the toddler will display a lack of interest in others and experience decreased communication skills.

Toddlers need consistency. Praise for accomplishments, no matter how small the feat, will build self-confidence and a willingness to keep trying new things.

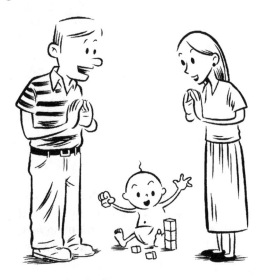

"GOOD JOB, DANNY. THAT'S
A NICE TOWER."

Therapeutic approaches in the medical setting include setting an example for parents to follow in response to the child's development. Many pamphlets, brochures, and books are available to help parents encourage early childhood development. Communication with toddlers is important, and interest should be shown in them as individuals. Converse on their level of understanding and always remember to be honest with them. If a procedure is going to be uncomfortable and the child asks if it will hurt, explain the process in terms understandable to the child. Tell how it will feel: the injection will hurt like a bee sting or it will feel like a pinch. Toddlers have fantastic memories and will recall if you have been dishonest at one time or another.

School-age children experience a great deal of stress as they begin the transitional activities between home and school. Suddenly the security of everything known to the child is shaken. When children feel threatened, they often revert to a more infantile behavior; this is called **regression**.

(See Appendix B.) Examples of such behavior include bed-wetting, thumbsucking, or stuttering. Other signals of stress during this time period are nail-biting, nightmares, a decreased appetite, headaches, and stomachaches.

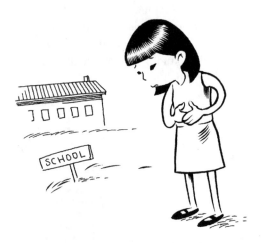

"OH, MY TUMMY HURTS."

To reduce stress for school-age children, suggest that parents discuss the activity well in advance. If possible, suggest a visit to the school, meeting the teacher, taking a ride on a bus, and showing the child where he/she will be met after school.

Adolescence is defined as a period of change. The body is in the process of changing from child to adult. With these changes comes stress. The development of breasts, narrowing of the waist and widening of the hips, growth of axillary and pubic hair, hormonal changes, and menstruation are some changes females experience. Males begin to broaden through the shoulders and develop upper body strength; facial, axillary, and pubic hair grows. They may experience acne, hormonal changes, and a cracking voice. Growth spurts make them awkward and clumsy.

Adolescents experience social demands and peer pressure as well. They are still children, yet in many ways are considered men or women. They are expected to make decisions regarding college and career goals, and they often begin their search for a mate.

Therapeutic approaches in the medical setting include providing privacy and modesty. Be sure to give plenty of time to disrobe. If possible, provide a drawer or dressing room closet where their clothes may be placed. Knock before entering the room. Understand that the primary concern of the adolescent is "How will this procedure affect my appearance or level of activity?" Teens fear being different in any way. Be honest and explain the procedure or process in terms they can understand. Respond to their questions and give them choices whenever possible.

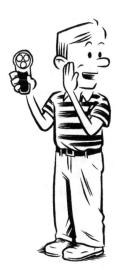

"THAT'S WHAT I CALL A CLOSE SHAVE."

Adults experience a variety of stressors. Mortgage payments, career commitments, and perhaps marriage and a family are just a few. Often adults are overloaded with too much to do and not enough time to do it. Many adults find themselves experiencing the "sandwich syndrome." Today's trend is to begin a family later in life, with many adults becoming first-time parents at the age of 35 or 40. This means their children are still under their roof when they begin to have responsibility for aging parents. They are caught in the middle, or sandwiched, between the two generations. Teenagers and aging parents both require intense energy expenditures and create many stressors.

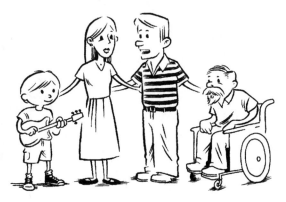

THE SANDWICH GENERATION
FAMILY

Adults also experience the "empty nest syndrome." The children are raised and off to college, or married and establishing their own homes. If the children have been their entire focus, parents may be stressed or depressed.

Adults often experience occupational stress or burnout. Some warning signs of burnout include withdrawal from others, negative feelings toward others, increased absences from work, and less efficient and effective approaches to work-oriented tasks. Irritability toward fellow employees, emotional outbursts, frustrations, and lack of self-control may also be exhibited.

Adults cope with stress better when they have a network of friends and/or colleagues with whom they can share. It is always helpful to know that others are experiencing similar feelings, and to learn how they are coping with them.

Answer adults' questions in the medical setting. It is often helpful to present pamphlets for details, which may be read away from the office setting. Encourage the adult to talk about their feelings and fears.

Aging is a privilege that provides many experiences from which to draw in the future. The elderly also face many stressors. Among these are retirement, illness, and death. We think of adolescents as experiencing much change during their development. The elderly also experience much change, and with change comes stress. Much of an elderly person's stress comes from loss rather than gain. They are slowing down physically and mentally. The body deteriorates and wears out. The mind is not as alert and it is difficult to remember things that were once so important. There is a loss of energy, agility, beauty, and family togetherness. Retirement brings the loss of a job, perhaps other losses of security, finances, structure, routine, and relationships. The elderly experience the death of spouses, friends, and acquaintances.

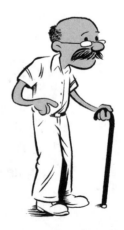

"SOME OF MY PARTS DON'T
WORK SO GOOD."

In the medical setting, there are several important steps that can be taken to decrease stress for the elderly. It is important to answer all questions. Encourage a family member to come along if there is important information to be given, or write down the instructions for the elderly. When addressing the elderly, use the person's full name and title, when appropriate. Encourage them to talk about accomplishments and express an interest in the elderly as individuals. Allow the elderly to make decisions regarding personal health care whenever possible, and use techniques that will foster self-esteem, dignity, and a sense of worth.

HOW TO REDUCE STRESS

Reducing stress can have an impact on your overall physical and emotional health. Migraines, high blood pressure, allergies, lower-back pain, depression, and ulcers have all been linked to stress. Here are some suggestions for reducing stress.

1. Any sustained aerobic activity, such as running, jogging, or dancing, relaxes muscles and also causes the body to release **endorphins**, naturally produced chemicals that can relieve stress and bring about a sense of well-being.

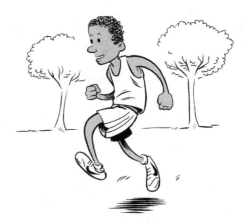

"JOGGING REALLY RELIEVES MY
STRESS AND GIVES ME A NEW
PERSPECTIVE ON LIFE."

2. Breathe deeply to feel tranquil. Stress causes quick, shallow breathing that increases tension. By taking deep breaths from the abdomen, you relax and increase oxygen levels to the brain.

3. Take a walk. Whenever possible, go outside and walk. Breathe deeply, stand erect, and walk briskly. When high-pressure situations arise in the office or at home, leave the room until you can calm down.

4. Limit caffeine and alcohol. These raise blood pressure and increase muscle tension.

5. Plan ahead. Whenever possible, rise and shine 15 minutes earlier in the morning. Get to meetings early and be prepared.

6. Let off steam. When all else fails, express your feelings privately. Cry into a pillow, punch the couch, stomp your feet, walk, run, or punch a punching bag.

7. Laugh. A hearty laugh is very therapeutic and relieves stress.

8. Pay attention to nutrition. A balanced diet and regular meals help reduce stress. Too much junk food and unbalanced meals are harmful.

9. Meditate. Silently repeat a favorite word, phrase, or verse.

10. Catnap. Taking a 5- or 10-minute nap can rejuvenate and reduce stressed nerves and muscles.

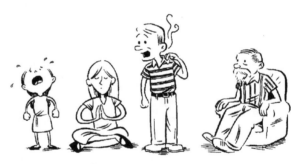

"EVERYBODY DEALS WITH STRESS DIFFERENTLY"

STOP AND CONSIDER

Review the opening case study at the beginning of this chapter. Now respond to the following questions.

1. What symptoms of stress did Janice demonstrate in this scenario?
2. What symptoms of stress did David demonstrate?
3. How did Janice decrease stress for David while they waited for 911 to respond?

THE THERAPEUTIC RESPONSE

- *Be honest with the client.* When the client asks questions, respond truthfully. Knowing what to expect helps the client understand their illness.

- *Offer educational materials.* Most health care facilities have access to excellent printed material related to various illnesses and diseases. There are also many Web sites that provide excellent information. Understanding the illness can empower the client to handle and prepare for outcomes.

- *Encourage emotional support.* The love and belonging level of needs within Maslow's Hierarchy of Needs is extremely important to clients experiencing stress. (See Appendix A.) Encourage clients to seek comfort and support from family, friends, specific support groups, spiritual groups, and community services.

- *Be a teacher.* Some clients or their primary caregivers may need to learn basic medical skills: for example, how to give an insulin injection or how to use percussion to help clients expectorate mucus from the lungs.

- *Provide community resource materials.* Have a list of community resources available to give to clients who may need additional support. Meals on Wheels can provide daily hot meals. Housecleaning services, skilled nursing facilities, and hospice and/or respite care are available in most communities.

ANXIETY

Internal stressors are created in the mind and are sometimes classified as "emotional allergies" or anxieties. **Anxiety** is a feeling of apprehension, worry, uneasiness, or dread frequently accompanied by physical symptoms, much as in the fight-or-flight stage. Anxiety is different from fear in? that fear is the reaction to a known and usually external threat. Anxiety, on the other hand, may occur at any time, develops from within, and may be triggered by any situation. There are four levels of anxiety: mild, moderate, severe, and panic.

Mild Anxiety

Mild anxiety is healthy, as it increases perception. During mild anxiety, our body functions well. It is stimulated by the increased production of adrenaline, which enables us to think clearly and focus on details; to be alert, organized and efficient; and to make wise decisions and judgments.

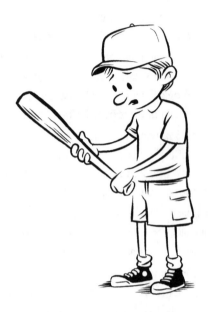

"WHAT IF I STRIKE OUT?"

Therapeutic responses to the person experiencing mild anxiety include providing details for health care, providing instructions, and offering choices regarding treatment when decisions must be made.

Moderate Anxiety

The person experiencing moderate anxiety has decreased perception. Their focus is on a particular task or problem rather than on the overall circumstance. When experiencing moderate anxiety, the individual will still be alert and able to think clearly. Concentration, however, will be focused on one challenge at a time. Decisions and judgments will be made on each individual detail as it is experienced or as the person becomes aware of another detail.

Physiological changes that may be noted during moderate anxiety include perspiration, increased heart and respiratory rates, and muscle tension. Gastrointestinal and urinary tract distress may also be experienced, causing frequent urinations and/or diarrhea. Behavioral manifestations may include irritability, pacing, inability to concentrate, and insomnia.

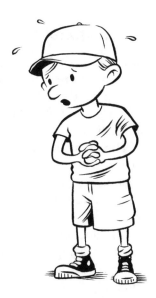

"I DONT' KNOW WHAT TO DO."

Therapeutic responses include focusing on one detail at a time; speaking in a soft, calm manner; encouraging relaxed breathing techniques; and keeping the person informed regarding how much longer the procedure will take or the time when the discomfort will be over. Sometimes just saying "You seem very anxious today" will help the person let go of some of the stress.

Severe Anxiety

During severe anxiety, individuals experience an inability to focus on details, or they may be able to focus attention only on one aspect of a situation. Abstract thinking is lost. Some concrete directions may be followed, but learning generally does not take place. Because of the inability to concentrate, these individuals will be very indecisive.

Physiological changes during severe anxiety include dry mouth, profuse sweating, rapid and shallow pulse and respiration, increased blood pressure, headache, speech impairment, increased muscle tension, and tremors or shivering.

Behavioral manifestations include purposeless movements, crying, confused communication, and an inability to think abstractly.

Therapeutic responses to severe anxiety include giving detailed instructions to a family member or writing out the instructions for the client. Give them brochures or pamphlets to read after they have had time to gain self-control. Telephone them later in the day or the next day to see how they are doing or if they have any questions.

Panic Anxiety

During the panic anxiety stage, individuals are consumed with escape. They want to remove themselves from the situation. Attention is focused on a minute detail that is often blown out of proportion. Speech is usually incoherent and communication ineffective. See Chapter 6 for additional information.

The physiological changes experienced during the panic stage are the same as those during the severe stage, but magnified. A prolonged state of panic can have serious consequences, even fatal ones. Behavioral manifestations are also the same as severe-anxiety-stage manifestations, only—again—greatly magnified.

Therapeutic approaches for panic anxiety are the same as for severe anxiety. It is important not to allow a person in this state to leave the office until recovery has taken place or until someone else can drive the person home.

SUMMARY

Stress is part of life, no matter what age group a client is in. Stressors signal the body to go into alarm, and may be caused by anything—fear, worry, threat, or even challenging events. Eustress helps the body function efficiently, make judgments and decisions, and work at peak performance. Distress may be harmful to the body, and is related to the intensity and duration of the stressor. During periods of distress, we are not able to function efficiently, make judgments and decisions, or work at peak performance.

Anxiety is a feeling of apprehension, worry, uneasiness, or dread frequently accompanied by physical symptoms, much as in the fight-or-flight stage of stress. Anxiety develops from within and may arise in response to perceived or real events. Levels of anxiety range from mild to panic anxiety, with each level impacting the ability to focus on details, concentrate, and to make decisions and judgments. Physiological changes during anxiety may also be noticed, with the increased production of adrenaline that occurs.

Health care professionals who understand human growth and development issues will be able to recognize stressors in their clients no matter what their age. Age-appropriate therapeutic responses will encourage the client to verbalize their feelings and concerns. Being able to suggest ways to manage or reduce stress is also helpful for the client.

EXERCISES

Exercise 1

Briefly describe your therapeutic response to the following situations. These exercises can be used in small group settings or can be completed independent of others.

1. Your client presents at the dentist's office experiencing moderate anxiety and is consumed with only that particular problem.
    Your therapeutic response includes_____

    _____

    _____

2. A new mom brings her infant to the pediatrician for his 6-week checkup. Both appear very stressed.
    Your therapeutic response to the mom includes_____

    _____

    _____

    Your therapeutic response to the infant includes_____

    _____

    _____

3. Fourteen-year-old Kenji arrives for his scheduled appointment. He appears very shy and nervous, and finally tells you he came because of his acne.
    Your therapeutic response includes_____

    _____

    _____

4. Your client and his wife arrive at the ambulatory care office because Alex thinks he is having a heart attack. After seeing the doctor, he is diagnosed with panic anxiety.
    Your therapeutic response includes_____

    _____

5. Rachael is very upset because the school nurse told her daughter Ty that she had scoliosis. Rachael made an appointment with the chiropractor for a complete examination, including X-rays.
    Your therapeutic response to Rachael includes_____

    _____

    _____

Your therapeutic response to Ty includes_____

_____

_____

Exercise 2

Using the Internet, look for self-help, bulletin boards, or other electronic reference sources that could help you, family members, or clients understand and manage stress. Make a list of the resources you have found to be shared with the class.

Exercise 3

Using Appendix A, review the age groups as discussed by each theorist. Identify potential stressors for each age group. Now, write a therapeutic response for each stressor listed.

REVIEW QUESTIONS

Multiple Choice

1. Hans Selye's General Adaptation Syndrome theory proposes that adaptation to stress occurs in how many stages?

   a. 2 stages

   b. 3 stages

   c. 4 stages

   d. 5 stages

2. Mild anxiety

   a. may include physiological changes such as perspiration, and increased heart and respiratory rates.

   b. may include behavioral manifestations such as irritability and pacing.

   c. may include inability to focus on details or focusing on only one aspect of a situation.

   d. is considered healthy because it enables one to think clearly, focus on details, and to make wise decisions and judgments.

3. During panic anxiety, therapeutic responses

    a. that provide details and instructions for health care are appropriate.

    b. include giving detailed instructions to a family member or in writing to the client.

    c. include keeping the client informed.

    d. include offering choices regarding treatment decisions.

4. Ways to decrease stress include all of the following *except*

    a. aerobic activity.

    b. planning ahead and being organized.

    c. mediation.

    d. enjoying caffeine or alcohol often.

5. Eustress is a term used to describe

    a. bad stress.

    b. anxiety.

    c. panic anxiety.

    d. good stress.

FOR FURTHER CONSIDERATION

1. How can health care professionals help the caregiver living with chronic stress while caring for an elderly parent with Alzheimer's 24-7?

2. How do men and women respond differently to stress? Give specific examples.

3. How does understanding human growth and development aid the health care professional to assess and deal with stress and the life cycle?

CASE STUDIES

Case Study 1

Elizabeth, a 68-year-old woman, has experienced relatively good health for most of her lifetime. A year and a half ago, she suffered a bout of pneumonia, with a very difficult recovery. She continued to "feel sick," and had no appetite. Weight loss and decreased energy levels ensued. Her primary care physician admitted her to the hospital for further tests, which revealed a diagnosis of Chronic Obstructive Pulmonary Disease (COPD) (although she had never been a smoker), and pulmonary aspergillosis. She was discharged with a PICC (peripherally inserted central catheter) line and daily administration of antibiotics at the IV therapy center. After three months of IV therapy, the aspergillosis seemed to be gone and Elizabeth felt somewhat healthier.

Houseguests visited Elizabeth during the summer, and one of them came down with a cold. With permanent damage from the COPD, a weakened immune system, and the trauma and stress that Elizabeth had just been through, she caught the cold, which developed into another bout of pneumonia. The aspergillosis returned and a pulmonary embolism and blood clot were found in her left leg. The PICC line was reinserted and Coumadin prescribed. This treatment meant daily trips to the IV therapy center and a stop at the hospital to have Coumadin levels evaluated.

1. What indicators of stress do you see manifested in this case study?

2. How can Elizabeth better deal with this stress?

3. How can health care professionals help her manage the stress?

Case Study 2

Juan is 3½ years old when a new sister joins the family. At first Juan is excited about having a new sister, because family members bring him presents and he also gets to open gifts brought for his sister. But when she cries, Mom is prompt to attend to her needs and Juan has to wait until his sister is settled before Mom can help him. Juan thinks it takes a long time for his sister to get her bath and eat her meals. He becomes frustrated at not receiving all of Mom's attention and begins to act out by shouting and sometimes throwing toys. Juan, who has been toilet trained for some time, begins to soil his pants and wants to drink from a sippy-cup again, rather than using his grown-up plastic cup.

1. What steps can his mother take to decrease Juan's stress and frustration?

2. According to Erikson, which stage of development is Juan experiencing?

3. What defense mechanism is Juan demonstrating? (See Appendix B.)

RESOURCES

Frisch, N. C., & Frisch, L. E. (2006). *Psychiatric mental health nursing* (3rd ed.). Albany, NY: Thomson Delmar Learning.

Mandleco, B. L. (2004). *Growth & development handbook: newborn through adolescent*. Albany, NY: Thomson Delmar Learning.

Milliken, M. E. (2004). *Understanding human behavior* (7th ed.). Albany, NY: Thomson Delmar Learning.

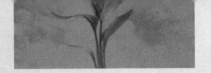

CHAPTER

6

THE THERAPEUTIC RESPONSE TO FEARFUL, ANGRY, AGGRESSIVE, ABUSED, OR ABUSIVE CLIENTS

CHAPTER OBJECTIVES

The learner should strive to meet the following chapter objectives and demonstrate an understanding of the facts and principles presented in this chapter through written and oral communication.

- Define key terms as presented in the glossary.
- Describe the behavior of a fearful client.
- List and describe three phobias.
- Discuss panic attacks.
- Discuss three therapeutic approaches to a fearful client.
- Describe an angry client.
- Identify at least five therapeutic approaches to the angry client.
- Describe the aggressive client.
- List at least four descriptors of inappropriate aggressive behavior.
- Describe the process created by anger, aggression, and verbal abuse.
- Discuss therapeutic approaches to the aggressive client.

- List at least four characteristics of an abuser.
- Discuss the three phases of violence.
- Recall four types of abuse.
- Define three types of violence toward others.
- Identify what constitutes
  - Intimate partner violence (IPV)
  - Child abuse and neglect
  - Elder abuse and neglect
- List the three categories used to identify rapists.
- Explain the crisis stages experienced by rape survivors.
- Discuss the many indicators of abuse.
- Recall treatment protocol for abused individuals.
- Explain documentation and reporting guidelines for instances of abuse.
- Discuss therapeutic responses to both the abuser and the abused.
- Examine personal attitudes toward fear, anger, aggression, and abuse.

OPENING CASE STUDY

A 36-year-old woman dressed in a high-powered suit and carrying a briefcase hurriedly approaches the pharmacy counter in a large national-chain drug store. The professional behind the counter (a pharmacy assistant) is caring for a customer at the drive-up window.

Customer: (clears her throat loudly) "Excuse me, but I need a prescription filled, and I am in a hurry."

Pharmacy Assistant: "I'm almost finished here. The pharmacist has stepped out for just a moment; he will assist you as soon as he returns."

Customer: "What do you mean, the pharmacist isn't here? Can't you help me?"

The pharmacy assistant, now finished with the drive-up window customer, looks at the prescription and says, "We can have this filled for you in 15 minutes."

Customer: (now clearly agitated) "Fifteen minutes! I haven't got all day. I came here, to this discount drug store, because I thought you would be faster than my regular pharmacist. I had to wait 45 minutes on the doctor, and now I have to wait on you. I will never make my afternoon appointment. Just throw those damn pills in a bottle and tell me what it costs."

Pharmacy Assistant: "Sorry, I can't do that."

Customer: "Then give me back my prescription; I'll go someplace where I can get some service."

Pharmacy Assistant: (tosses the prescription back at the customer) "Good riddance."

The pharmacist returns just as the customer storms away and says to him, "Fire that incompetent witch."

STOP AND CONSIDER

1. Identify the stressors the customer exhibited.
2. At what point did the stress become anger?
3. What happened to the pharmacy assistant to cause her to respond as she did?
4. How would you describe the actions of the customer?
5. What would you have done in the same situation?

INTRODUCTION

The therapeutic response implies that the health care professional will be relating to people in need. Often these people will be fearful, angry, and even aggressive. Sometimes they are abusive or abused.

Recognizing and understanding such behavior enables the professional to more easily respond in a therapeutic manner.

THE FEARFUL CLIENT

> ## ❧ CASE STUDY ❧
>
> *Harry, a 49-year-old construction worker recuperating from a myocardial infarction, returns to the medical office for a follow-up evaluation. Harry is uncooperative; Dr. Cooper discovers that Harry is not taking his anticoagulants, is back to work a month prior to the recommended time, and is still chain-smoking. Harry is more concerned during this visit about his sex life than he is about the serious consequences of his behavior.*

Fear is an emotion aroused primarily by something you are uncertain of or by some sort of threat, whether real or imagined. There are different degrees of fear, and fear varies with each individual. Fear can lead to social problems if not appropriately addressed. Fear has many definitions, but some are distrust, worry, dread, fright, paranoia, or terror. *Distrust and worry* are emotions that usually focus on a person or object. The fear is gone when the person or object disappears. For example, when a client is fearful of a blood draw, distrust of the laboratory technician and worry about the discomfort can induce fear. Once the blood is drawn, the bandage in place, and the client leaves the area, however, the fear subsides. *Dread* is the fear usually experienced prior to an event. A client who shrinks back when a nurse approaches the hospital bed with a syringe in hand knows what is coming and dreads the event. *Paranoia* is a psychosis of fear that is related to a feeling of being victimized. Paranoia can cause irrational or compulsive behavior. Women who have been unsuccessful in getting pregnant and who are desperate to give birth to a child may break down in uncontrollable sobs when they discover that another menstrual period has begun. They wonder why this happens to them. *Terror* occurs when an individual is overwhelmed with a feeling of impending danger. This kind of fear may cause an illogical reaction. The woman who cannot get pregnant may rebuff all sexual contact with her spouse, believing that it doesn't make any difference anyway; she will only fail again.

Fear and/or fright are exhibited in many ways. Physiologically, the client may have sweaty palms, experience a fast heartbeat, feel a temperature change in the body, and have a sinking feeling in the pit of the stomach. Children exhibit fear easier than adults. Many adults are so conditioned by comments such as "There is nothing to be afraid of" that they may hide their fear. In the adult population, fear is often denied, hidden, or masked by other behavior. This *suppression* (Appendix B) may eventually turn into *somatic* symptoms.

A client's denial of fear may be an unconscious *defense mechanism*—an attempt to protect oneself by blocking an emotionally painful experience. People using this mechanism are unable to recognize the cause of their discomfort and may even deny being frightened or fearful. Some clients can be so threatened by their illnesses that they will not permit themselves to be aware of their feelings. These clients tend to be hypercritical of treatment and unusually demanding. It is difficult for these clients to accept help from their caregivers, since to do so is to acknowledge their fears.

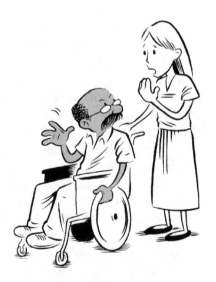

"BUZZ OFF. I CAN DO IT."

Often fearful clients will not cooperate in their treatment regimen. This is exhibited in the case study on p. 127. For Harry to recognize the possible consequences of a myocardial infarction and to take appropriate action, he would also have to accept his fear.

Panic Attacks

Intense fear, sometimes known as *phobia*, daily impacts the lives of some individuals. Three common phobias are acrophobia, claustrophobia, and agoraphobia. **Acrophobia** is the fear of high places, and **claustrophobia** is fear of being confined in any small space. **Agoraphobia** is a fear of public places, and usually develops after having one or more panic attacks. It is the fear of being alone in a public place where there is no easy escape if a panic attack occurs. Symptoms of a panic attack may include dyspnea, sweating, vertigo, palpitations, chest pain, nausea, dread, and even the feeling that there will be a loss of control. When panic is intense, there can be a feeling of approaching death. Panic attacks may last up to an hour and often leave a client feeling exhausted. These fears are abnormal when they interfere with daily living activities or when they cause an individual to take extreme measures to avoid the feared experience.

Not much is known about the cause of phobias and panic attacks. There may be some connection between phobias children have and the phobias their parents have. Medications alone or medications combined with behavior therapy have been successful in treating phobias and panic attacks.

THE THERAPEUTIC RESPONSE

It is important to *recognize and accept the client's fears.* Statements such as "This can be very frightening" help a client feel accepted even though fear has been exhibited.

The *problem-solving approach* often reveals an acceptable solution. Once the client visualizes a solution, the fear begins to decrease.

In the opening case study at the beginning of this chapter, fear might have been dispelled had the pharmacy assistant said, "It seems you are quite concerned about being late for your afternoon appointment. Would you like to leave the prescription now and come back after work to pick it up?" This offer might have reduced the fear felt by the woman, if she could visualize making her appointment as well as having the prescription filled.

Allow the client as much control over the situation as possible. When clients feel in control of the treatment, they are less fearful. Explain procedures and treatments carefully, taking time to assure clients and allay their fears. A client can feel fear even if they have an extensive medical background.

continues

The Therapeutic Response continued

Act for the client who is panic-stricken. Such people are unable to act for themselves and need the assistance of another. For instance, a person listening to her best friend's panic over a lump in her breast may pick up the phone to make an appointment with a physician for her friend, and also go with her to the appointment. When panic occurs in the health care setting, stay with the client until the panic subsides. If appropriate, explain the situation to the partner or friend who may accompany the client.

THE ANGRY CLIENT

❧ CASE STUDY ❧

James approaches your desk to make another appointment. He is obviously agitated. He slaps a piece of paper on the counter. You recognize it as a diet the physician has prescribed for his diabetic condition. He sarcastically says to you, "It is impossible to stay on this diet! Who does that doctor think she is?"

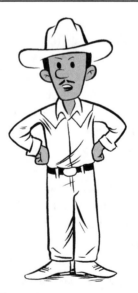

"WHO DOES THAT DOCTOR THINK SHE IS?"

Anger is another emotion that may be brought on by fear, threats, obstacles, or offensive situations. In most cases anger is temporary, and is often directed toward a specific object or person. *Annoyance* is a term used to describe a mild form of anger, and *resentment* is a chronic form of anger that is long lasting. Intense anger or animosity directed toward a particular person or people is termed *hatred*. Any form of anger that is not resolved may have a negative impact on one's behavior after an extended period.

Inappropriate expression of anger includes hostility that is displaced or physically acted out against another person. Such anger can lead to injury or harm to another person. (See *displacement* in Appendix B.) Hostility is displaced when it is directed toward someone or something other than the cause of the frustration. If a person is angry over circumstances at work and takes it out on the family cat, this is displaced hostility. Anger that is not properly managed easily turns into aggression.

Every human being experiences anger. What is done with anger is the key to a healthy mental attitude. Anger can generate positive energy. If the emotion encourages an individual to find a solution to a problem, change an unhealthy lifestyle, or manifests itself in appropriate physical activity, the anger is not turned inward to breed contempt or cause physical ailments later.

Clients who are angry are usually easy to recognize. They have an angry tone in their voice and in their facial expression; they are apt to use profanity. Generally, they talk rapidly and rarely listen. Angry clients usually feel frustrated and annoyed. The frustration can come from any number of sources and may or may not be correctly addressed to the health care professional. Janet's frustration, in the previous case study, may be over a diet she cannot follow because 1) she likes little or none of the foods, 2) she is afraid she cannot follow the diet, 3) she is afraid she's losing control over her life, or 4) she is dealing with some totally unrelated incident in her life.

Health care professionals will, from time to time, experience angry comments made by clients. To understand and cope with these comments, some recommendations follow.

THE THERAPEUTIC RESPONSE

- *Do not take offense at a client's comments or take them personally.* Evaluate the actions on their merit, not as a personal affront. This requires control and a healthy self-esteem on the part of the health care professional.

- *A demanding client may really be lonely, anxious, frightened, or insecure.* Give reassurance and offer explanations of services or procedures. Try to determine what the client really needs and work toward a solution.

- *Accept clients as they are.* Help your clients regain their self-esteem by talking out their angry feelings. "You seem quite upset about this new diet" is a comment that

continues

The Therapeutic Response continued

encourages Janet to tell more about her hostile feelings, but does not make her feel ashamed.

- *Use techniques to de-escalate client anger.* Speak in a calm, reassuring voice, and at a slightly slower pace than usual. Use controlled expressions. Let the client know that anger is an appropriate emotion, but gently indicate what you will not be able to accept.

- *Be patient and do not rush interactions.* Allow clients to express their anger in a controlled, unhurried atmosphere. Often, just being able to verbalize frustrations calms an individual who is angry. Once the client is calm, return to a solution to the problem without further mention of the anger.

- *Listen carefully to verbal and nonverbal communication.* Remember the communication cycle. The message may have to be decoded and checked for its validity to determine the real message. Health care professionals may find it difficult to listen because they are anxious to defend their position.

- *Do not defend or blame.* Do as much as possible to help resolve the problem. Do not argue with the client; to do so will only escalate the situation. Any defense also heightens the anger of the client. If you are unsuccessful in calming the client, call for assistance.

- *Document everything.* Carefully document the entire episode completely. In doing so, remain neutral regarding your feelings. Describe the incident, what was said, and how you responded. Identify any actions taken to resolve the conflict. Be very careful not to use derogatory language in your documentation. It is not appropriate, for example, to say, the client was "rude." State facts, not emotions.

- *If you find yourself feeling hostile toward clients,* examine your feelings and discuss your response with someone who can help you sort through your reaction. Continuous giving to others can drain you, but you must be relatively free of anxiety to be therapeutic.

- *Take a breather* following an upsetting episode with a client. Even a few minutes can help calm your own feelings and enable you to give full attention to your responsibilities. Take a coffee break, walk around the block if you can, perform some other task for a few moments. All of these examples can help to ease stress and anxiety.

THE AGGRESSIVE CLIENT

If conflict escalates beyond the angry state, clients may become aggressive and/or verbally abusive. In the opening case study, the verbal abuse occurs when the customer and the pharmacy assistant belittle each other and make threats. The pharmacy assistant's "Good riddance" statement while tossing the prescription back at the customer escalates the customer's anger into additional verbal abuse and aggression when she says to the pharmacist, "Fire that incompetent witch."

Some individuals have an underlying aggression that only exhibits itself when control is lost. This kind of aggression usually is the result of unresolved anger and a loss of self-esteem. Some descriptors of people exhibiting aggression inappropriately include the following:

- becoming suspicious of others over very small matters

- joking at someone else's expense

- confronting people with long, involved analyses of their behavior

- becoming hostile, antagonistic, or resentful, or carrying a grudge

- becoming uncooperative, caustic, sarcastic, rude, and critical

- becoming demanding, complaining, and/or threatening

- threatening to inflict or actually inflicting personal injury

Although you can do little about a client's unresolved anger, it may help to recognize that unresolved anger may be a possible reason for aggression. Helping clients cope with anger and aggression is important. If aggression is turned inward on self, the client may become depressed. Both children and adults need to be taught appropriate behavior for dealing with their anger.

Sometimes it is difficult to know when conflict may turn to aggression and verbal abuse, but it is for certain that, when anger is not diminished and the conflict intensifies, aggression and verbal abuse are likely to follow. It may help to remember that the expressions of anger, aggression, and verbal abuse move through a process illustrated below:

Physical or Emotional STRESSOR

↓

Painful FEELINGS

↓

ANGER

↓

ACTING OUT

The customer in the pharmacy was stressed because she had to wait in the doctor's office and she feared the possibility of missing an important engagement. She is likely feeling inadequate, since she believes she will fail to make the appointment. This is a painful feeling. These feelings lead to the statements that express frustration. The pharmacy assistant may not have encountered someone like this before, but feels responsible for "fixing" the problem. (A good question to ask in such a situation is, "Is it my responsibility to 'fix' this problem?")

Trigger words or statements are a response to the painful feelings. Triggers come from one's own values, beliefs, or expectations about how things should be. Anger follows, then acting out.

THE THERAPEUTIC RESPONSE

The guidelines for a therapeutic response to clients who are angry are also important to remember for clients who are aggressive. It is always better to try to resolve the conflict, placing yourself in the shoes of the other person to understand their needs and frustration, yet protecting yourself as necessary. Setting personal limits is helpful. "I can call another pharmacy with this prescription for you, if you cannot wait a few moments. Otherwise, I will ask you to leave if you continue to swear at me and make threats." This kind of statement alerts the offender that the limit has been reached. Often the offender will become embarrassed and retreat rather quickly. Then an agreeable solution is quite possible.

If the client continues to threaten and the anger increases, protect yourself. "I cannot accommodate your needs. Please leave the pharmacy now." Most individuals will leave. If not, make certain you have an escape route. Move yourself closer to the door. Call for assistance. This action may shock the aggressor into quieting down.

As a helping professional, you must remember that you chose this profession. You made a conscious decision to serve people. You daily enter into relationships with your clients that are *nonreciprocal*. If clients become angry and belittle you, you do not have the right to belittle them back. You have the right not to lose your self-respect, but you do not have the right to disrespect your clients. You must always remember that your client is worthy of respect, no matter how wrong he or she is. The respect you give your clients is not dependent upon their achievements or lessened by their inappropriate behavior.

continues

The Therapeutic Response continued

With those thoughts in mind, the best way to respond to angry, aggressive, and abusive clients is to listen empathically, show respect for others and yourself, remember not to take the event personally, and communicate assertively as necessary. Do not let someone else's bad day ruin yours. Learn how to short-circuit the anger process. Consider the following statements as possibilities:

- "It must be frustrating to have to wait, first for the doctor, and now for the pharmacist."

- "While I cannot fill this prescription for you, I can hasten the process by getting everything started for the pharmacist. Do you have insurance? Is this a medication you have taken before?"

- "Here's the pharmacist now. I will tell him you are in a hurry."

- "Would you like to use our phone to call your appointment while we get the medication ready?"

- "Thanks for choosing our pharmacy. I hope your afternoon goes a little more smoothly."

ABUSED OR ABUSIVE CLIENTS

✤ CASE STUDY ✤

Sam is brought to the medical office by his granddaughter and primary caregiver, Rebecca. Rebecca always comes with her grandfather, but seems agitated and nervous on this visit. Sam is suffering from the first stages of senile dementia. In the examination room, as the medical assistant rolls up Sam's sleeve to take his blood pressure, she sees large black and blue blotches on his skin. She asks, "Sam, what happened here?" Sam replies in a whisper, "Rebecca hits me when I soil the bed."

In the previous section, you learned about how anger is processed and how it escalates. Turn your attention now to abusive behavior that is acted out toward individuals—many times in the family setting, and often to those who are powerless to change the actions of the abuser. This type of abuse may be emotional, physical, or sexual. Abusive behavior may come from friends and acquaintances, family members, and less often, strangers. Behavior is *violent* when there is intent to do harm. This harm may be in the form of emotional abuse, which is at first less obvious than physical or sexual abuse. In general, abuse is usually the result of biological, psychological, social, and cultural factors.

STOP AND CONSIDER

Before reading further, gather your thoughts about abuse and abusive relationships.

1.   What are you feeling?
2.   Have you known someone in a relationship that is abusive?
3.   How do you feel about someone who abuses another?

Abusers usually suffer from low self-esteem and feelings of powerlessness, and blame others for their actions. They are also angry and frustrated. Without a feeling of self-worth, it is difficult to be confident and assertive; therefore, people with low self-esteem and a lack of confidence have a difficult time maintaining close and intimate relationships. They often feel threatened. Violence becomes a way to gain power and control over others.

Abusers are manipulators, and easily rationalize and minimize their abusive behavior. They find it much easier to blame others for their abusive behavior than to accept responsibility for themselves. Abuse most often occurs when people have not been able to control their feelings of frustration and anger. The smallest event can trigger an abusive episode. The people closest to the abuser at this time usually become the abuser's target.

PHASES OF VIOLENCE

Violence has been identified in a number of ways, but the three phases of violence most often used to describe abuse are 1) the tension phase, 2) the crisis phase, and 3) the calm phase. These phases may vary depending upon the individuals and the particular circumstances; sometimes the phases do not exist at all. When they do exist in an abusive situation, the phases are likely to become shorter, more violent, more frequent, and increasingly unpredictable over time.

Tension Phase

There may be a triggering event that precipitates this phase. Tension builds; communication breaks down. It may be the 4-year-old spilling milk all over the dinner table, or an adult getting into a "fender-bender." The abuser begins to lose control and humiliates the abused with verbal attacks. The abused often tries to placate or appease the abuser in order to cope. As the verbal assaults continue, threats are made. Pushing or slapping may occur. The abused will try to avoid the abuse; the abuser blames the abused for the situation. The abused often becomes detached emotionally and psychologically as the abuser increases control and possessiveness.

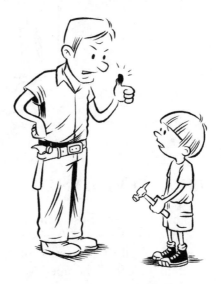

"CAN'T YOU DO ANYTHING RIGHT?"

Crisis Phase

As anxiety reaches a climax, the abuser is very unpredictable; a series of "minor" assaults may occur over a period of time, or there may be very serious injury from a major assault. Death can even result. This phase may last just minutes or several hours. The abuser may isolate or lock up the victim. The abused will try to adapt in order to survive, and may even escape, but usually returns after the crisis is over.

Calm Phase

The abuse ceases. The abuser may ask forgiveness and be very loving; however, the abuser will continue to blame the abused. Both the abuser and the abused are relieved the crisis is past. Both may be emotionally and physically exhausted. The abused wants to believe that the violence will not happen again.

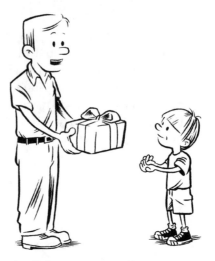

"I'M SORRY ABOUT WHAT HAPPENED. IT WON'T HAPPEN AGAIN."

TYPES OF ABUSE AND VIOLENCE

Four types of abuse will be covered in this chapter. They are intimate partner violence (IPV), child abuse, elder abuse, and rape. At one time or another, all health care professionals will be faced with the challenge of communicating therapeutically with both the abusers and the survivors of such abuse.

Intimate Partner Violence (IPV)

Intimate partner violence (IPV) is defined by the Centers for Disease Control and Prevention (CDC) as physical, sexual, or psychological/emotional violence directed toward a spouse or former spouse, current or former partner, or current or former dating partner. IPV refers to abuse between married people or people in an intimate heterosexual or same-sex relationship. The term *domestic violence* may be used, also; however, intimate partner violence defines the broader scope of the problem. The abuser may be either male or female. Some authorities add stalking to the definition of IPV. **Stalking** is the repeated behavior that causes individuals a high level of fear, and may refer to actions such as following, spying upon, pursuing, and threatening.

The violence described in the CDC's definition of IPV fits in other areas of abuse, also, but is further defined here.

Physical Violence

This type of abuse uses physical force with the intent to do harm. There is the potential for injury, disability, even death. Physical violence includes, but is not limited to, choking, shaking, throwing, pushing, scratching, punching, burning, using a weapon, restraining, and using one's body size and strength against another.

Sexual Violence

Sexual violence includes 1) forcing a person to engage in a sexual act against his/her will, even if the act is not completed; 2) attempting or completing a sexual act with an individual who is unable or incapable of understanding or declining participation in the act because of disability, the influence of alcohol or drugs, or intimidation; 3) abusive sexual contact.

Psychological/Emotional Violence

This type of abuse may include, but is not limited to, humiliation and control, isolation from friends and family, withholding information, deliberately embarrassing or diminishing the individual, and denying access to resources.

The last decade has seen an increase in reports of intimate partner or domestic violence. Survivors of this type of abuse often report living in relationships characterized by fear, anger, and frustration. Wife battering is most commonly reported, but husband battering is on the rise. Women may receive more serious injuries since, generally, they have less physical strength than men, but women are more likely to use a weapon when they abuse.

In some cultures women continue to be viewed as property—first of their fathers, then of their spouses. This patriarchal authority, still supported by some religions, leads some men to believe that their wives must submit to their authority or be disciplined by them. Abused women often rationalize that their abuse is caused by their own behavior and their own worthlessness. It is interesting to note that a person who leaves an abusive relationship or divorces the abuser still mourns the death of the abusive relationship. To obtain emotional health, this individual may need to work through the grieving process.

Child Abuse

Child abuse is evidence of parental/caregiver frustration, anger, and inability to fulfill parental obligations. Some parents and caregivers envision a fine line between discipline and abuse, and child abuse statistics are inadequate in describing the problem. Many individuals are reluctant to report child abuse even when mandated to do so by law. Few family members will admit to abusing or neglecting their children, and children usually do not admit they have been abused. Many think the actions against them are normal or are the result of some wrong they have committed. Children's sense of self comes from the parents or primary caregivers who are abusing them.

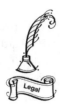

The 1990 Victims of Child Abuse Act defines abuse and neglect in the following terms: *Child abuse* refers to the deliberate harm or injury of a child by a parent or caregiver. *Negligence* occurs when a parent or caregiver fails to provide the basic necessities for life. *Physical injury* refers to serious bodily harm, severe bruising, lacerations, fractures, and internal injury. *Mental injury* includes harm to a child's psychological or intellectual well-being. *Sexual abuse* involves coercing a child into sexually implicit conduct, including molestation, rape, prostitution, or any form of sexual exploitation. *Sexually explicit conduct* is actual or simulated sexual intercourse, masturbation, lustful exhibition of the genitals, or sexual gratification from inflicting pain on others. *Child molestation* involves oral-genital contact, genital fondling or viewing, and masturbation. *Sexual exploitation* is child prostitution or pornography where sexually explicit reproductions of a child's image are used. *Incest* refers to sexual relations between children and blood relatives or family members.

People who abuse children sexually often were sexually abused themselves. Abusers may begin to abuse in their teens. If discovered, the excuse of experimentation will often dismiss their offenses. Most sexual abusers will repeat the behavior throughout their lives, even when caught and punished or given treatment. There is no reliable method of changing the behavior of people who sexually abuse children.

The close parent-child or primary caregiver-child relationship often confuses health care professionals trying to make a diagnosis, since both parties will exhibit deep concern for each other. Parents or caregivers who bring abused children in for treatment are often careful never to use the same clinic twice, and always have an explanation for the injuries.

Elder Abuse

Elder abuse is defined as the harm or neglect that is inflicted upon someone who is 60 years of age or older. Elder abuse is more under-reported than child abuse. Identifying abuse of the elderly is difficult unless there is outright battering. Even then, excuses are likely offered. The abused elderly rarely report violence toward them, mostly because they fear loss of a living arrangement or retaliation. The elderly are also ashamed that someone they may have nurtured in childhood is now abusing them.

Elder abuse most likely occurs in two locations: 1) in the home or primary living residence of the elderly person (domestic elder abuse), and 2) in a nursing home or some type of long-term care facility (institutional elder abuse). Elder abuse occurs in many different forms:

- *Physical abuse* is identified as threats or harm that result in injury, impairment, or pain. Physical abuse includes, but is not limited to, beating, whipping, slapping, pushing, shoving, shaking, kicking, pinching, force-feeding, inappropriate use of drugs or restraints, and any rough handling.

- *Psychological/emotional abuse* occurs when there is a lack of basic emotional support, respect, and love. This type of abuse includes name-calling, verbal assaults, and dehumanizing the elderly. It may include isolating the person from family and friends, threatening to punish, intimidating, treating the elder person like a child, and terrorizing.

- *Neglect or abandonment* consists of confinement, denial of essential needs, or isolation. The neglected elder may lack the necessities of food, water, shelter, clothing, medicine, warmth, and safety. Individuals may not have adequate assistance with bathing, be physically restrained, lack assistance in moving around their environment, and have lack of access to supplies for incontinence. Abandonment occurs when a caregiver deserts a vulnerable elder adult.

- *Sexual abuse* is sexual contact without consent. Sexual abuse may include kissing, fondling, or touching of the genitals or making the elderly person fondle someone else's genitals. Sexual assault or forcing the elderly to observe sexual acts or pornographic material is sexual abuse. Telling "dirty" stories, spying on the elderly in the bathroom, and forcing nudity upon the elderly is sexual abuse.

- *Financial exploitation* is the use of finances, property, or anything of value belonging to the elder in an illegal or improper manner. Any misuse of the elder's belongings, such as withholding Social Security checks, using a charge card without permission, scamming or tricking the elder person into withdrawing money from the bank and then taking the money, stealing household goods or valuables, forcing an elderly person to alter a will to benefit the abuser, and forging the elder adult's signature are considered financial exploitation or abuse.

- *Violation of rights* includes denial of adequate medical care, taking property without due process, not allowing the elderly person to attend religious services of his/her choice, and taking away a person's right to make their own decisions while they are still competent to do so.

Institutional elder abuse may occur in any of the forms just described. There are other violations, however, that may occur in a long-term care setting. The use of physical restraints may be necessary on rare occasions; however, when restraints are applied against the elderly person's will or the wishes of family members because of understaffing or lack of training, or when the staff is too busy to pay adequate attention to an elderly person, institutional abuse occurs. Other forms of institutional abuse are over- or under-medicating, force-feeding, rough handling while moving the elderly or giving medications or treatment, ignoring pleas of help, improper hand washing by health care providers, inadequate attention to changing diapers or disposable briefs, failing to provide adequate psychological care or stimulation, overcharging or double-billing for medical or personal services, and stealing personal property or money.

Caregivers in nursing homes and long-term care facilities may be inadequately educated, trained, and prepared for the task. Often they are not comfortable with the language or culture of the elderly, and if serious disease or dementia is involved, it is far less stressful to treat the elderly individual as a nonperson. It is fairly easy to provide simple care for the elderly, but it can become far less pleasant if the caregiver must feed, bathe, and provide assistance in the bathroom. If the elderly is appreciative of the care and is able to communicate, the caregiving is made easier. If the elderly person is aggressive, even violent, the caregiver will be more stressed, and may struggle to remain professional at all times and in all situations.

Caregiving in the home is very stressful, also. Caregivers may be overburdened with the responsibility of caring for an older adult. This may cause the caregiver to ignore the basic needs of the elderly. Often, younger caregivers do not understand the social needs of the elderly. They do not realize that the losses (significant other, driver's license, physical health, etc.) suffered by the elderly precipitate grief. The despair, complaints, and criticism expressed by the elderly who are grieving may become difficult for the caregiver to understand or tolerate.

Psychological and physical changes associated with aging may cause some older people to withdraw from social activities. Caregivers may tire of sitting and listening to these elderly people. They assume the role of parent and assign the role of child to the elderly person. This role reversal discourages the older person's independence and integrity.

Rape

Rape is forcible sexual intercourse with an unwilling partner. The rape incident may include *sodomy*. Rape is not a sexual act. It is an act of violence. No person invites rape, either by behavior or dress. Rape may include more than one person or more than two, as seen in gang rape. *Criminal sexual assault* is identified as penetration of any part of the abuser's body with any object, using force and without consent. Anyone can be raped: infants, the elderly, lesbians, gays, people with disabilities, and individuals of every ethnic, social, religious, and cultural background. While the majority of rape is committed against women and girls, men and boys are raped also. Men and boys are often attacked by gangs and are assaulted with weapons.

Law enforcement personnel and many legal professionals refer to the individual who has been raped as a "victim." Most health care professionals and social service professionals refer to the individual who has been raped or abused as a "survivor." Words and their meanings are very powerful. Both words will be used in this text.

Health care professionals may find it helpful to recognize that rapists are generally identified in three categories: angry, power, and sadistic. The *angry rapist* displaces anger to the abused, uses a fair amount of physical force, and degrades the victim by forcing oral sex or masturbation. The angry rapist may urinate on the victim. The angry rapist most often preys on someone who is older or vulnerable.

The *power rapist* is the most common type, and uses only the amount of force necessary to subdue the victim. The power rapist is seeking power and control and often intimidates the victim. The power rapist may fantasize that the victim is sexually attracted to the rapist, wants to know if the victim "is enjoying this," and may ask to see the victim again after the rape.

The *sadistic rapist*, the least common type, seeks sexual gratification as an outlet for aggression. Sexuality and aggression go hand in hand. This rapist is aroused by the victim's death, and may achieve orgasm at that moment. Penetration may be obtained with an instrument. The rapist may have intercourse with the victim after death.

Survivors of rape generally experience four distinct crisis stages in their recovery. They are as follows:

- The first phase is one of shock, disbelief, and fear. This phase can last for two to three weeks in some cases.

- The second phase is a time of adjustment. The survivor may appear outwardly to be doing fine, but inwardly is in denial of the entire event.

- The third phase is a time of depression, self-doubt, and the need to talk about the rape. Often, the survivor has difficulty sleeping and is quite anxious.

- The fourth phase is a time of recovery, with the recognition that the blame lays totally with the abuser rather than the survivor. The survivor begins to trust others again and feel comfortable in daily activities.

Like any experience that may be described in phases or stages, survivors do not necessarily go through all the stages in a given pattern. They may go through the phases many times, or may never move out of one phase. How clients cope is dependent upon factors such as how others react to the event, their own personal development, and their willingness to participate in crisis counseling. The latter allows the opportunity for support and the ability to discharge the shame, guilt, and anger felt over the event.

INDICATORS OF ABUSE

Emotional abuse is often not evident until many years later. Emotional abuse usually takes its toll in long-lasting physical or psychological problems and is difficult for health care professionals to diagnose. However, health care professionals should be aware of those who are often extremely punitive in their treatment of others, who are aggressive and verbally abusive to others, and who are easily threatened by others or exhibit a low self-esteem. Individuals who have been abused typically have few defense mechanisms for coping with anxiety and stress. Health care professionals can and should provide resources to help them learn to control their abusive behavior.

Physical abuse may be observed by health care professionals when survivors seek medical attention or are brought to health care facilities by family or friends. Burns, bruises, lacerations, broken bones, malnutrition—all are examples of what may be physical evidence of abuse. Special attention should be given to the individual who denies any form of abuse when the abuse seems obvious. It is important to provide survivors with information on how to keep safe, help survivors realize that they were not the cause of the abuse, and allow them their personal dignity.

Children who are physically abused will exhibit evidence of the abuse. X rays may reveal fractures in various stages of healing. Burns, bruises, and lacerations are often apparent. Sexual abuse may be evidenced by difficulty in walking or sitting; torn, stained, or bloody underclothing; pain or itching in the genital area; bruises or bleeding in external genitalia, vaginal, anal, or mouth areas; and sexually transmitted diseases (especially in preteens) or pregnancy. If medical treatment is sought early enough, rape or sexual intercourse may be evidenced by the presence of semen. In some cases, there may be no obvious physical signs or symptoms.

Children who have an interest in or knowledge of sexual acts or language inappropriate to their age may have been sexually abused. These children may reenact sexual scenes with dolls, in drawing, or with friends. They may attempt to touch the genitals of adults, other children, or animals.

People who are physically abused may exhibit aggressive behavior, and children also may *regress* (Appendix B) to an earlier stage of development, such as wetting or soiling their underwear. Children may threaten their playmates or dolls. People may be aggressive toward animals, and anger is directed everywhere. Abused people often withdraw into a fantasy world. People may exhibit fear of specific places or people. Sleep disturbances and nightmares are common.

TREATMENT

Any abused individual coming to a health care facility must receive prompt treatment for any injuries. A rape kit must be done immediately in cases of rape. A rape kit is filled with little boxes, microscope slides, and plastic bags for collecting and storing evidence such as clothing fibers, hairs, saliva, or semen.

Samples of this evidence may be used in court. The circumstances and the place of treatment will determine if law enforcement is notified at that time. The survivor needs to feel safe and have a safe place to go. Provide a list of such places or other possible resources, and discuss alternatives. Focus on the survivor, not on the violent event. Underlying anxiety and anger needs to be assessed. The survivor needs acceptance and approval and is very vulnerable to any form of rejection, real or perceived. Eventually, survivors must be helped to confront the crisis and talk about their feelings. Survivors need to identify effective coping behaviors to deal with the crisis. Community agencies may provide the best resources for this process.

Remember that abusers also need treatment. Health care professionals treating an abuser must be assured of a safe environment for themselves and the abuser. Observing the abuser's personal space is important, so as not to appear threatening. A violent person may have a personal space requirement up to four times larger than for a nonviolent person. Involve the abuser in therapy; it is helpful if the courts require therapy. The abuser must learn assertive, nonviolent ways of expressing anger and frustration and communicating with others. Try to communicate acceptance of the abuser's feelings but *not* acceptance of the violent behavior.

REPORTING AND DOCUMENTATION

All states have laws that identify specific requirements for reporting abuse. All 50 states mandate the reporting of child abuse. IPV is a criminal offense in some states, but not all require reporting unless a weapon is used for the abuse. A majority of the 50 states have enacted legislation regarding elder abuse. It is not the purpose of this text to be a legal guide, since new laws are legislated almost daily; therefore, health care professionals must become knowledgeable of their state's requirements. Hospital and emergency room personnel are generally more equipped to report, document, and treat an abused individual than the ambulatory health care professionals. However, not all abused individuals present themselves to emergency rooms.

Each state has laws defining child abuse and mandating that suspected child abuse and neglect be reported. People most likely required to report suspected abuse and neglect include health care professionals, social service and law enforcement personnel, educators, and professional people working with children. Any person who believes that a child may be abused or neglected may report, in good faith, to law enforcement or child protection agencies. Such people are protected against liability as a result of making the report, provided there is reasonable cause to suspect child abuse or neglect. Reports may be made by telephone, in writing, or in person to the local law enforcement agency or appropriate state agency.

The most difficult circumstances may be when an abused elderly adult or a survivor of IPV asks that no report be made to law enforcement officials. If states do not have laws that mandate reporting the offense, protecting the survivor from further abuse may be the best approach. Make certain these individuals have the telephone numbers of safe places to go and that they understand their options.

The health care records of survivors of violence and abuse will likely be used in a court of law. The medical record should not, therefore, include inferences or conclusions of the assault. Only facts should be reported. Those facts might include

- history and account of the incident
- words expressed by the client(s) and in quotations
- photographs of injuries when possible
- documentation, if known, of the extent of force that was used
- specific, factual observations
- objective findings and treatment established

Any evidence collected (body fluids, clothing, etc.) is to be bagged, labeled, and safely preserved and protected for law enforcement, making certain the "chain of evidence" is not broken. Anyone reporting the case should write down the information as clearly and completely as possible.

THE THERAPEUTIC RESPONSE

Some suggestions are made under "Treatment." (See p.145.) Responding therapeutically in any circumstance involving violence and abuse is a challenge. It helps to concentrate on the individual seeking treatment and not on the violent act. Do not shame or ridicule. Be gentle, calm, and supportive. Give reassurance and offer explanations of the services and procedures. Be patient and do not rush interactions. Note the nonverbal as well as the verbal responses of the client. Assure the client's safety, privacy, and prompt treatment. It is important to assist both the abuser and the abused to seek proper counseling. This may involve personal as well as family counseling. Parents Anonymous provides support for parents who have abused their children. VOCAL (Victims of Child Abuse Laws) assists people who have been falsely accused of child abuse. There are support groups for IPV survivors and rape victims, also. They include VOICES: Victims of Incest Can Emerge Survivors; RAINN: Rape Abuse Incest National Network; and a number of Web sites related to IPV available on the Internet.

Unless a trust relationship already exists between health care professionals and the abuser or the abused, it may be difficult to establish therapeutic communication.

It is interesting to note that survivors usually experience the same kinds of feelings as the abuser. Their self-esteem may be seriously damaged by the abusive situation. They feel powerless and often blame themselves. They feel ashamed, frustrated, and angry. They grieve the loss of their self-concept. Significant others and family members pose problems if

continues

The Therapeutic Response continued

they are not supportive and accepting of the victim. Health care professionals can assist family members and friends in understanding this dimension of abuse and recovery.

One of the goals in any of the violent situations identified is to protect survivors from any further abuse and to break the cycle of violence. Individuals may need temporary shelter. Always have a list of phone numbers available for such services. Encourage family members to seek counseling and treatment. Help potential abusers identify their tendency toward abuse and seek treatment. Provide appropriate rehabilitative and supportive services to high-risk families. Survivors of abuse can get caught in multiple social agencies that have differing goals. Clients easily become confused and even feel victimized again by the actions taken to protect their abuser. Encourage these clients to hold fast to their goals and continue the path to recovery.

UNDERSTANDING SELF

It is important for health care professionals to examine their own attitudes toward fear, anger, aggression, abuse, and the abuser. Treating these clients with disgust, anger, and avoidance is not a therapeutic response. Stereotypes about individuals who are easy to anger, become aggressive, or inflict violence need careful self-assessment. Feeling frustrated and powerless to change situations of long-standing abuse can prevent a therapeutic response. A health care professional who lives in a household where anger and aggression is commonly expressed or who has witnessed abuse may have difficulty in remaining objective and being helpful to either the abuser or the abused. But the opposite also may be true. Health care professionals who have "traveled down the same path" may be the most therapeutic because they know what is and is not helpful.

It can be difficult to respond therapeutically to clients who are angry, or who get aggressive, even abusive, in their response to you as a health care professional, and it is even more difficult to respond therapeutically to the abusive client. Personal feelings that enter into the relationship cloud a professional's effectiveness unless they can be set aside.

SUMMARY

Health care professionals who are therapeutic realize that their roles may place them in circumstances that can be frightening, unpleasant, even revolting, and that they will be called upon to perform their duties with sensitivity and without judgment. Health care professionals who are successful in this task lead a balanced daily life and see the potential for good they can bring to all situations. They have learned how to set limits and how to be compassionate without emotional attachment, and they have learned to recognize their vulnerabilities. They understand the nonreciprocal relationship between client and health care provider.

EXERCISES

Exercise 1

1. Identify at least three facilities in your community that would be appropriate resources for the client who may be experiencing fear or aggressive behavioral patterns.

2. Discuss with a close friend how you and the members of your living group (family, dormitory roommates, etc.) deal with expressions of anger and aggression.

Exercise 2

Respond to the following situations:

1. Dick, a businessman who has been waiting for his appointment for 20 minutes, says, "I'll not wait another moment for the doctor. Please recommend another physician who can see me."
    You feel_____.
    You respond_____.

2. Sharon, a coworker, remarks to you, "Why do you always insist on making such a mess in the appointment schedule?"
    You feel_____.
    You respond_____.

3. You must tell the client who is smoking in the lobby that he cannot smoke in the hospital. How will you explain that policy?

    _____.

    _____.

4. The doctor angrily thrusts a medical chart under your nose and says, "Where are the lab slips that should have been in here a week ago?"
    You feel_____.
    You respond_____.

Exercise 3

Select a character who is an abuser or a survivor of abuse in a novel, movie, or television program. What kind of behavior characteristics do this person exhibit? Write a short report with your response.

Exercise 4

Briefly describe what you would say and how you would respond to the following situations. These exercises can be used in small group settings or can be completed independent of others.

1. Your spouse/significant other uses verbal abuse and inappropriate language when you are arguing.
    I feel _____.
    I would say _____.

2. Your date does not listen or respond when you say "No" and "Stop" during hugging, kissing, and fondling.
    I feel _____.
    I would say _____.

3. A stranger approaches who makes suggestive remarks.
    I feel _____.
    I would say _____.

4. Assume you have just been a victim of physical and sexual abuse.
    I feel _____.
    I would want health care professionals to say

    _____.

    What would have to happen for you to feel like a survivor rather than a victim?

    _____.

REVIEW QUESTIONS

Multiple Choice

1. Identify the statement that is untrue.

    a. Physical fear is usually long in duration.

    b. Panic fear is intense and may be immobilizing.

    c. Fear is an emotion aroused by uncertainty or threat.

    d. Fear is often denied and hidden, and can cause somatic symptoms.

2. Panic attacks

   a. may cause dyspnea, sweating, and vertigo, and interfere with daily activities.

   b. may be treated with medications and behavior therapy.

   c. rarely last more than 15 minutes.

   d. a and b above are correct.

3. Abuse

   a. may be emotional, physical, or violent.

   b. comes mostly from strangers.

   c. is a way to gain power and control over others.

   d. is often identified in four phases.

4. The three phases of violence are

   a. the calm phase, the trigger phase, and the crisis phase.

   b. the tension phase, the crisis phase, and the calm phase.

   c. the trigger phase, the verbal phase, and the unpredictable phase.

   d. the trigger phase, the tension phase, and the violent phase.

5. Intimate partner violence (IPV) refers to physical, sexual, or emotional abuse from

   a. a parent or former parent.

   b. a spouse or former spouse.

   c. a current or former partner or dating partner.

   d. b and c above.

6. Elder abuse

   a. is defined as harm or neglect inflicted upon someone 55 years of age or older.

   b. most likely occurs in the home, in a nursing home, or in a long-term care facility.

   c. is better reported than child abuse.

   d. a and b above.

7. Rape is

   a. not a sexual act.

   b. an act of violence.

   c. forcible sexual intercourse with an unwilling partner.

   d. a, b, and c above.

FOR FURTHER CONSIDERATION

1. Discuss with an acquaintance the use of the term *survivor* rather than *victim*. Can you identify circumstances where one term is preferred over the other?

2. The term *intimate partner violence* is often used instead of *spousal abuse* or *domestic violence*. Discuss the meaning of each and identify when one might be preferred over the other.

CASE STUDIES

Case Study 1

You are a certified nursing assistant sitting with another assistant at break time in the lounge. Your morning has been particularly frustrating, but you are surprised when your colleague blurts out, "I can handle the dementia people most of the time, but when they get mean, I get mean right back!"

- What do you say? What do you do?

- Identify any suggestions you might make to help your colleague.

Case Study 2

You are in a department store with your spouse and teenage son. You are all aware of a fairly noisy gentleman who approaches the counter, asking where he might find boys' pajamas. A woman who appears to be his wife and a young boy are with him. The man notices sweatshirts with humorous slogans on them. One women's sweatshirt says, "The Queen Who Must Be Obeyed" on it. He jerks his son by the arm, points to the sweatshirt, and says, "We don't have that kind of b_ _ _ in our house, son, and you won't have that either!" The woman looks at you with pleading eyes, but shrugs her shoulders and walks away.

- What kind of discussion might you have when your family returns to the car?

- What information is important for your son to have?

RESOURCES

Domestic and dating violence handbook (2002). Seattle, WA: Metropolitan King County Council.

Frisch, N. C., & Frisch, L. E. (2006). *Psychiatric mental health nursing.* Albany, NY: Thomson Delmar Learning.

Lewis, M. A., & Tamparo, C. D. (2007). *Medical law, ethics, and bioethics* Philadelphia, PA: F. A. Davis Company.

Purtilo, R. B., & Haddad, A. (2002). *Health professional and patient interaction*. Philadelphia, PA: Saunders.

Saltzman, L. E., Panslow, J. L., McMahon, P. M., & Shelly, G. A. (2002). *Intimate partner violence surveillance*, (version 1.0.). Atlanta, GA: Centers for Disease Control and Prevention, National Center for Injury Prevention and Control.

Schuster, P. M. (2000). *Communication*. Philadelphia, PA: F. A. Davis Company.

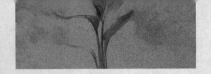

CHAPTER
7

THE THERAPEUTIC RESPONSE TO DEPRESSED AND/OR SUICIDAL CLIENTS

CHAPTER OBJECTIVES

The learner should strive to meet the following chapter objectives and demonstrate an understanding of the facts and principles presented in this chapter through written and oral communication.

- Define the key terms as presented in the glossary.
- Differentiate between the following types of depression and identify each type's signs and symptoms.
  - minor depression
  - major depression
  - reactive depression
  - endogenous depression
  - involutional (melancholia) depression
  - dysthymic disorder
  - unipolar depression
  - bipolar depression (BPD)
  - seasonal affective disorder (SAD)

- postpartum depression (PPD)
- substance-induced mood disorder
- Discuss the impacts of depression upon the life span.
- Identify a minimum of four therapeutic approaches to depressed clients.
- Identify the high-risk groups for suicide.
- List the steps and stages involved in contemplating suicide.
- Differentiate the verbal and nonverbal messages sent by suicidal people.
- List criteria used to evaluate suicide potential.
- Identify a minimum of five therapeutic approaches to the suicidal person.

OPENING CASE STUDY

Recently Jody, a 15-year-old, has not been acting like herself. She used to hang out with her friends after school; now when she comes home, she goes straight to her bedroom or stares at the television for hours. Jody was a very good student; however, her teachers report that she does not turn in assignments on time and her test scores are dropping. When asked about this, Jody responds, "I don't care. What's the point of it all?" When her friends call, she does not want to talk with them. She was active in her church youth group, but now is not interested in participating in their activities. She seems tired and listless and has lost noticeable weight. When her parents try to talk to her about what is wrong or how she feels, she gets irritable and snaps at them. She seems angry with them for expressing concern. Jody states, "I can't do anything. Everything I want is hopeless and I'm worthless. Why bother?" This has been going on for several months, and her parents wonder if something is seriously wrong.

INTRODUCTION

Depression has been described as feelings of despair, gloom, or emptiness; a sense of foreboding, numbness, hopelessness, or agony; or a negative sense of self-worth. Anyone can experience depression, and it can be brought on by a number of different causes. People may become depressed when their feeling of well-being is challenged or when they experience a loss of some type. Others experience depression because of unpleasant feelings, including sadness, boredom, apathy, even anger.

Signs and symptoms vary, depending upon the type of depression experienced. They may cry for no apparent reason, be quiet with very little to say, and may even shy away from friends and family. Sleeping and eating patterns may be disrupted, causing additional fatigue and restlessness.

There is no diagnostic test for depression, such as a blood test or scan, which is able to confirm whether someone has the illness. In the past, different psychiatrists used different criteria to diagnose depression. With the advent of internationally recognized sets of diagnostic criteria such as the **Diagnostic and Statistical Manual (DSM)** and the **International Classification of Disease (ICD)**, much confusion has been alleviated. These criteria have led to a greater uniformity of approach to the diagnosis and classification of depressive illnesses. The criteria and the classes of depression are constantly updated with each new revision of DSM and ICD, and there continue to be differences in opinion between psychiatrists.

Researchers believe all depression involves some changes in brain chemistry, even when the cause of depression is clearly a psychological trauma. After psychological treatment and recovery from depression, the brain chemistry returns to normal, even without medication. Many respond to treatment better when psychotherapy is provided in addition to medication. Medication treats the symptoms of depression; however, the psychological problems that caused the depression must also be addressed.

More than 32 million people in the United States will experience a major depressive disorder in their lifetime. This happens regardless of gender, race, ethnicity, or income. Some interesting facts include the following:

- Depression is among the leading causes of disability worldwide.

- Women are nearly twice as likely as men to experience depression.

- People with a family history of depression may be more likely to develop the disease.

- People with chronic or debilitating medical conditions may also be susceptible to the disease.

- A major life change, even a joyous one like becoming a new parent, increases the risk of developing depression.

TYPES OF DEPRESSION

Two types of depression are defined: minor and major. Primarily, the intensity and duration of the symptoms, and the specific cause of the symptoms are used to diagnose depression. Types of depression are termed **clinical depression** when symptoms are severe enough to disrupt the client's daily life and treatment is required.

Minor Depression

Minor depression is a lesser-used term for a subclinical depression that does not meet criteria for major depression. For those who almost always seem to have symptoms of a mild form of depression or who have intermittent symptoms, the diagnosis is dysthymia or minor depression.

Dysthymic disorder is characterized by a chronic, low-level depression that lasts for a minimum of two years. These clients feel depressed almost daily and may progress to a major depression when a crisis occurs. The depression causes changes in thinking, feeling, behavior, and physical well-being. Changes in thinking include problems with short-term memory, forgetting things all the time, and inability to concentrate. Negative thinking and pessimism are also common signals of dysthymic disorder. Examples of changes in feeling are lack of motivation and becoming more apathetic. These characteristics may lead to feelings of helplessness and hopelessness. Behavioral changes such as anger with temper outbursts, excessive crying, and decreased sexual desire may also be experienced. Physical well-being changes, such as chronic fatigue, decreased appetite, weight loss, and just not feeling well further complicate the client's ability to function normally.

Major Depression

Major depression is the most severe category of depression. In major depression, more of the symptoms of depression are present, and they are usually more intense or severe. An episode of major depression can result from a single traumatic event in one's life, or may develop slowly as a consequence of numerous personal disappointments or life problems.

According to the fourth edition of the *Diagnostic and Statistical Manual,* a diagnosis of major depression requires the presence of at least one major depression episode. The episode must 1) last at least two weeks, 2) represent a change from previous functioning, and 3) cause some impairment in a person's social or occupation functioning. Diagnosis also requires five or more symptoms, one of which must be either a depressed mood or a loss of interest in previously enjoyable activities.

Subtypes of major depression include reactive depression, endogenous depression, involutional (melancholia) depression, unipolar and bipolar depression (BPD), seasonal affective disorder (SAD), postpartum depression (PPD), and substance-induced mood disorder.

Reactive Depression

Reactive depression is also referred to as an adjustment disorder with depressed mood. It is considered the most temporary form of depression and often follows the loss/death of a family member, a divorce, loss of a job, or not getting an anticipated promotion. *Loss* is the key. The loss may also include the loss of love, beauty, a home—loss of anything with meaning to the individual.

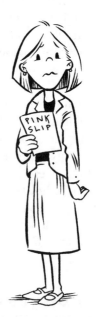

"THIS IS REALLY DEPRESSING."

Some signs and symptoms of reactive depression include 1) a decreased appetite and weight loss of under 10 pounds, 2) worsening depression as the day progresses, 3) difficulty falling asleep (DFA) and 4) slowing of body functions, causing urinary retention, constipation, and decreased hormone levels.

Usually individuals suffering from reactive depression are able to work through the emotional distress for themselves. Medications are not recommended, since time seems to reduce the situation. Family and friends can be a big support, as they may be aware of the precipitating factor. Sympathy and support in a person's time of need help the person resolve what has happened. Showing interest in the person's needs and listening to what is said are extremely therapeutic. Do not become intrusive, however; allow individuals to decide how much, and when, they wish to discuss the situation. Use your best listening skills. As you listen with the ear, observe with the eye any nonverbal communication cues. Encourage individuals to share their feelings. If they cry, remember that tears can be therapeutic, and will help relieve the sadness. Say something like, "I understand how difficult this time is for you. Crying sometimes helps in dealing with a situation."

Endogenous Depression

Endogenous depression comes from within and implies there is no discernible cause for the depression. Endogenous depression is cyclic, meaning that it occurs during particular life cycles or at the same time each year. The middle-age period is the most common life-cycle period, and Christmas or springtime are common times of the year for this form of depression. There also seems to be some link to familial tendencies, possibly biochemical in nature.

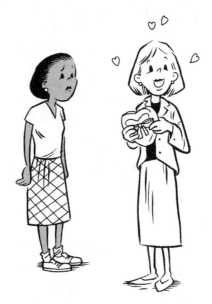

"THESE SPECIAL DAYS REALLY MAKE
ME FEEL SAD AND ALONE."

Symptoms include a substantial weight loss (greater than 10 pounds) and a feeling that the depression came on gradually and out of the blue with no precipitating event. Early morning awakening is often experienced with feelings of worthlessness. However, the symptoms may improve as the day progresses. Endogenous depression tends to be time limited, that is, the depression tends to run its course.

Mood elevators are the treatment of choice by most physicians. It is important to explain the dosage and any side effects. Many of these medications will change the color of urine. Alert the client to this possibility to avoid adding to the stress level. These drugs also have a lag time, or delayed therapeutic effect. That is, individuals may need to take the medication for up to three weeks before they begin to notice the effects.

Involutional Depression (Melancholia)

Involutional depression usually occurs during middle age or later. Women between the ages of 40 to 55 and men 50 to 65 years of age represent the target group. The personality of individuals who experience involutional depression is often described as rigid, overconscientious, and emotionally unstable. There is usually no previous history of mental illness.

Signs and symptoms of involutional depression include 1) delusions of sin, guilt, or poverty; 2) obsession with death; and 3) agitation, irritability, and pessimism. The onset of the illness is slow, with an increase in **hypochondriasis** and delusions associated with an exaggerated **paranoid ideation**. These individuals present themselves to health care professionals describing any number of ailments and disorders. Often the symptoms described are subjective, not perceptible to the senses of another person. Negative results of diagnostic evaluations and/or reassurance by physicians only increase the feelings of anxiousness and depression. Individuals become suspicious and mistrust the diagnosis, so will seek help from another source.

The prognosis for untreated people with involutional depression is poor. Treatment with antidepressants or electroconvulsive therapy (ECT)—the use of electric current—has been found effective in this disorder.

Unipolar versus Bipolar Disorder

The difference between unipolar and bipolar disorder can only be determined over the course of the illness. In the case of **unipolar disorder** the client experiences solely episodes of depression. In the case of **bipolar disorder** the client experiences both depression and elation or mania. In many instances, the observation of both highs and lows in mood are not observed until well into the course of the illness.

Both unipolar and bipolar depression can be inherited. The children of unipolar affective disorder parents have an increased risk of this type of depression. The children of clients with bipolar affective disorder have an increased risk of both unipolar and bipolar disorders.

Bipolar Disorder (BPD)

Bipolar disorder (BPD), also known as bipolar disorder, manic-depression, and manic-depressive illness, alternates between the extreme highs of mania and the severe lows of depression. Every person with BPD has a unique pattern of mood cycles combining depression and manic episodes that are predictable once the pattern is identified. There seems to be a strong genetic influence as well. Typically, BPD begins in adolescence or early adulthood and continues throughout life.

Signs and symptoms during the low or depressed phase of the disorder may include a persistent sad, anxious, or empty mood with feelings of helplessness, guilt, or worthlessness. The client may be pessimistic, demonstrate a loss of pleasure in usual activities, and can be irritable or restless. They may experience sleep disturbances, with decreased energy and loss of appetite. Suicide may be contemplated.

During the manic phase of the disorder, signs and symptoms may include excessive "high" or euphoric feelings combined with sustained periods of unusual, even bizarre, behavior, with significant risk taking. They may demonstrate increased energy, activity, rapid talking and thinking, and agitation, and may be extremely irritable and easily distracted. They frequently show poor judgment, deny problems, and have an unrealistic belief in their own abilities. These clients may require little sleep and frequently show an increased sex drive.

Bipolar disorder treatment includes medication and psychotherapy. Psychotherapy helps clients cope with the cyclical nature of the disease and can lead to better compliance with bipolar disorder medication.

Medications for depression are used in two ways. The first way is to control symptoms that are out of control and need immediate attention. These medications are known as *acute phase medications*. They are used to treat severe depression or suicidal behavior during depressive episodes, and they help control dangerous, psychotic behavior that accompanies some manic episodes. First-line medications for the acute phase of bipolar disorder may include lithium, valproate, carbamazepine, lamotrigine, and olanzapine. These medications function to stabilize mood. Smaller dosages of these medications are used to prevent future episodes of mania or depression. When used for this purpose, these medications are known as *chronic phase* or *preventative medications*.

STOP AND CONSIDER

Review the opening case study about Jody and respond to the following:

1. List Jody's emotional symptoms of depression.
2. List Jody's physical symptoms of depression.
3. What action should her parents, teachers, and friends take?

Seasonal Affective Disorder (SAD)

As the winter months progress, daylight hours grow shorter, and winter storms fill the skies with dark clouds. These conditions will likely be severe for those who live in the northern parts of the world. The decreased sunlight causes some individuals to develop **seasonal affective disorder (SAD)**, considered a subtype of depression.

SAD afflicts about 5 percent of United States adults—some 10 million Americans—but an estimated 25 percent of the population experience some form of winter blues. Winter blues vary in severity from mild "winter blahs," to moderate "winter doldrums," to severe winter depression, medically known as seasonal affective disorder.

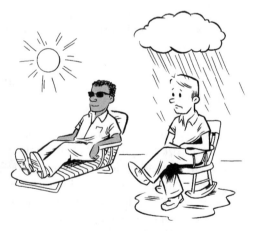

"MY GET-UP-AND-GO
GOT UP AND WENT."

Women with SAD outnumber men four to one. The disorder also strikes about 4 percent of children, and does seem to have familial tendencies. The symptoms of SAD include a noticeable decrease in interests normally pursued during the winter. Some say, "My get-up-and-go got up and went." They may experience as much as a 20-pound weight gain during the winter months. Signs and symptoms of SAD may include sleep disturbance, overeating (especially carbohydrates), depression, despair, misery, and anxiety. Family and social problems, irritability, antisocial behavior, and loss of sex drive may also occur. Physical symptoms may include joint pain, stomach problems, suppressed immune system, and lethargy.

Light therapy or phototherapy has become the treatment of choice for SAD. These individuals should get as much natural sunlight as possible. They may need to trim the bushes around windows or keep curtains and blinds open to allow more light to enter rooms. They should be encouraged to take walks, and to consider taking part or all of their vacation during the winter, visiting sunny areas of the country. As soon as spring arrives, the symptoms disappear.

Postpartum Depression (PPD)

Postpartum depression (PPD) is a severe form of "baby blues" lasting anywhere from three months to one year. About 10 percent of new mothers develop PPD. It is more common in women who have already experienced some form of depressive illness. Stress seems to be one of several contributing factors to this type of depression. A new mother can feel overwhelmed with the responsibilities involved with infants and small children. Sleepless nights, a colicky baby, illness, and lack of physical and emotional support for the new mom all add stress to this new family unit. When one adds the additional factor of fluctuating hormones and their role in postpartum depression, it is little wonder that many women experience this disorder.

Some mothers are afraid to admit they are depressed for fear of being deemed unfit or unable to care for the infant and perhaps losing it to social services. Support groups can play a major role in recovery. Sometimes just knowing that others also experience similar problems seems to be therapeutic. Physical and emotional support for an entire family can be found in support groups. Signs and symptoms of PPD frequently occur a few days after giving birth and include most of the symptoms found with other types of depression. Women suffering PPD frequently have experienced previous episodes of depression, and may have had a miscarriage or loss of an infant. They may lack support from the father or their family members.

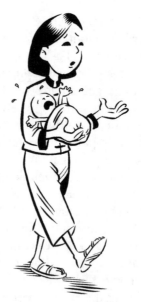

"WHY DOESN'T HE SLEEP MORE?"

Drug therapy can be helpful in some cases; however, caution must be used with the type of medication prescribed. Many medications enter the breast milk of nursing mothers and are passed on to their baby.

Substance-Induced Mood Disorder

A number of common prescription drugs have side effects that can create **substance-induced mood depression**. Pharmacies are required by law to include information about how and when a drug is to be taken, identify any side effects, and provide warnings such as "take with food," "may cause dizziness," or "do not operate heavy equipment." Examples of drugs with depressive side effects may include cardiac drugs and hypertensives, sedatives, steroids, stimulants, antibiotics, and analgesics. In most cases, once the offending medication is discontinued the depressive symptoms stop as well.

Often people self-medicate symptoms of depression with prescription, over-the-counter, illegal recreational drugs, or alcohol. Use of any of these self-medications to decrease depressive symptoms is more likely to increase the depression. Chemicals within the drugs or alcohol may actually cause clinical depression. Those with a chemical dependency and depression will have dual diagnoses. This simply means that the client has both an emotional disturbance and a drug and or alcohol problem, making recovery more challenging.

DEPRESSION AND THE LIFE SPAN

Depression will impact everyone at some time during the life cycle. The depression may be their own or that of a family member or acquaintance. Depressive disorders affect approximately 20 million American adults over the age of 18 in any given year.

Children

According to a study published in *Psychiatric Services*, April 2004,[1] preschoolers are the fastest growing market for antidepressants. At least 4 percent of preschoolers and 23 percent of older children are clinically depressed. Children experience the same symptoms of depression found in adults, and often with the same severity. Many times these symptoms are overlooked as normal or misdiagnosed for disorders such as attention deficit disorder (ADA) and attention deficit/hyperactivity disorder (ADHA). According to child development experts, depressive behaviors lasting beyond two weeks should be investigated.

Adolescents

Adolescents are at great risk of depressive disorders because of the many changes that they are experiencing. These changes include physical changes in the body and the emotional influences due to increased hormonal action. Often the family structure changes, adding to the stress, and peer pressure is an ever-present factor for consideration among teens. Some researchers suggest that stresses are dealt with differently by boys and girls. For example, boys are more likely to develop behavioral and substance abuse problems, while girls are more apt to become depressed. Depressive disorders are quite common among adolescents, with 8.3 percent suffering from some form of depressive disorder. About 7 percent of those commit suicide.

Adults

Women are almost twice as likely as men to experience major and dysthymic depression. This ratio does not seem to be influenced by racial and ethnic background or economic status. Men and women have about the same rate of bipolar disorder, although its course in women typically has more depressive and fewer manic episodes. About half of the adults who are depressed believe depression is a personal weakness and are too embarrassed to seek help. Women are more likely to admit to feelings of depression and seek professional help. Men, more often than not, are socially conditioned to deny these feelings and to bury them. As a result, men are more apt to "act out" when they are under stress, with a higher incidence of physical violence and higher rates of alcoholism.

Elderly

Elderly people do not adapt to change as readily as younger individuals. Often, the elderly are isolated from family and friends, who do not live nearby. The elderly have experienced more loss and grief. Previous coping methods used by individuals will have a direct impact on the individual's ability to adapt and accept change. If you know an elderly person who seems depressed, suggest a medical workup. Reassure them that depression is an illness and is fairly easily treated. Do not delay treatment until the elderly person begins to discuss suicide. Compared with younger people, the elderly talk about killing themselves less, but are more successful at the attempts. Fostering a sense of dignity, self-esteem, and value in the elderly will go a long way in preventing depression.

THE THERAPEUTIC RESPONSE

Individuals experiencing the effects of depression must have an environment in which they feel nonthreatened and secure enough to share their innermost feelings. Health care professionals should reinforce the client's ability to make personal decisions and problem-solve. When appropriate, it is helpful to include family members in the problem-solving process.

It is important to identify situations that arouse feelings related to unmet needs. Discussions that stimulate recall of past experiences and positive outcomes and coping methods are beneficial. Assist individuals in manipulating their environment so that they can effect change. Recognize that helplessness may be a learned response and provide situations in which clients can exert some control over their environments.

In response to behavior that indicates hopelessness, do not become "Suzy Sunshine" and try to talk clients out of their depression. Instead, work with them to develop experiences that will provide them with positive feedback.

When working with depressed clients some additional considerations include the following:

- Understand the disorder. Health care professionals need to research and learn more about depressive disorders in order to help clients understand, cope, and seek professional help.

continues

The Therapeutic Response continued

- Listen to clients. Health care professionals should encourage the client to discuss their feelings and listen in a nonjudgmental manner.

- Encourage the client to seek professional help.

- Provide access to community resources.

CASE STUDY

Marlene has made a decision. She has decided that her life is no longer worth living. She is making elaborate plans to end it. She calls her sister, Marti, and makes a date to meet her for a cup of coffee. While they are having coffee, Marlene gives Marti a manilla envelope with some personal belongings in it. When Marti opens it, Marlene comments, "It is just some things I want you to have if anything should happen to me."

SUICIDE

Statistics indicate that about 15 percent of the population will suffer from clinical depression at some time during their lifetime, and that 30 percent of clinically depressed individuals will attempt suicide. Half of them will succeed.

Suicide is the eighth leading cause of death for U.S. men, with half of all attempts involving firearms. Women attempt suicide three times as often as men; however, the success rate is only one-quarter that of men. For ages 15 to 24, suicide is the third leading cause of death. The elderly have the highest ratio of successful suicide attempts and in most cases have been seen by their primary care physician within weeks of the suicide attempt.

Four Stages of Contemplating Suicide

The individual contemplating suicide usually goes through the following four stages.

Stage #1

The individual's needs are not being met, so he/she becomes frustrated. Anger and hostility develop and the anger turns inward. Respond by trying to help the client identify needs not met and the source of the frustration.

Stage #2

A stress situation becomes unbearable and panic sets in. The individual begins to look for a means of escape or to mobilize help. Be a resource to this client and carefully listen to their concerns. Try to move them back to Stage #1.

Stage #3

In an effort to seek help, the individual will communicate his/her help-lessness to someone else. This is the point at which you can make a difference. Respond with care. Listen. Let the person know he/she is not alone. Keep in touch.

Stage #4

The individual then begins the suicidal process. The person cannot help himself/herself. The feeling is that no one else cares, so "I'll end it all." The person begins to develop a plan to carry out the goal, then makes the preparations to carry out the plan. If under a physician's care for depression, the person may call to have a prescription refilled. Next, the person carries out the plan by taking the whole bottle of pills at one time. Intervention may be the only appropriate response.

Danger Signs of Suicide

Most suicides do not occur without warning. By recognizing the signs that indicate someone may be contemplating suicide, and by taking these signals seriously and responding quickly, most suicides can be prevented.

Clients at high risk for attempting suicide include those with the following symptoms and common factors:

- *Previous attempts of suicide*: Between 20 and 50 percent of people who kill themselves have previously attempted suicide.

- *Depression*: Most suicidal people are depressed; know the signs and symptoms of depression and encourage treatment plans.

- *Situational risk factors*: Stressful life events such as the death of a loved one, recent loss of employment, and divorce are examples of situational risk factors.

- *Contagion*: Exposure to suicide or suicidal behavior by others is demonstrated by teenagers and young adults with suicide clusters.

- *Demographics*: Males are three to five times more likely to commit suicide than females. Most suicides occur among people less than 40 years of age; however, the Caucasian elderly population displays the highest rate of suicide.

- *Talking about death or suicide*: Over half of the suicide victims communicate their plans to someone before they follow through.

- *Planning for suicide*: Many victims will give things away, say their good-byes, put personal things in order, pay off debts, prepare a will, and make funeral arrangements.

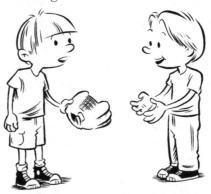

"I REALLY DON'T USE THIS VERY MUCH ANY MORE AND YOU ALWAYS LIKED IT. SO I'D LIKE YOU TO HAVE IT."

Communicating Suicide Plans

Over half of all suicide victims communicate their plans to someone before the attempt. They may use one of three approaches to communicate these plans.

- *Indirect*: "What would you do if I were not here to nag at you?"

- *Direct*: "I wonder what it feels like to die." Or "I wonder how it feels to die."

- *Coded verbal messages*: "I hate autumn—everything is dying."

Coded messages are nonpersonal—it is something else that is dying. Just as nonverbal communication must be read in clusters, so these cues must be considered in the context of other messages.

THE THERAPEUTIC RESPONSE

Prevention is the only significant intervention. Remember *every* threat or attempt of suicide is serious. This is a time to sit down, pull in close to the individual, and listen. Let the person know you really care, that you are a friend or professional, and that you will not leave or desert him/her. Tears are therapeutic, so cry if it is appropriate and you are sincere. Sometimes there is nothing you can do but sit in silence and perhaps hold the person's hand.

continues

The Therapeutic Response continued

Paul Welter, in his book *How to Help a Friend*[2], offers some therapeutic approaches.

- Listen.

- Do not give "pat answers" and easy advice.

- Make every effort to understand the mind-set of the person.

- Communicate through the person's strong learning channel—visual, auditory, or touch/movement.

- Avoid arguments and power struggles. As a helper, you need to help the person to become less perturbed, not more perturbed.

- Let yourself feel some of the other person's sufferings, and acknowledge the reality of their sufferings. By responding in an empathic way, you may come across as saying, "I care." This is sometimes an effective way to reduce the amount of self-hatred.

It is helpful to let the person know that you see the pain and agony they are going through and that you care. Encourage the person to talk about how he/she is feeling and why. Ask what you can do to help, and be sincere in your offer.

Have a list of appropriate referrals. When in doubt as to your actions as a health care professional, ask your employer. Do not wait, though. Time is important in potential suicide.

STOP AND CONSIDER

1. How does the Marlene scenario fit with the four stages of contemplating suicide?
2. How does Marlene communicate her helplessness to her sister, Marti?
3. How might Marti be therapeutic with Marlene?

SUMMARY

Depressive disorders impact many people regardless of gender, race, ethnicity, or financial status. Depression is the leading cause of disability worldwide, and can strike children, adolescents, adults, and the elderly. Creating a nonthreatening environment in which the client can express their innermost feelings, knowing that they will not be belittled or made to feel inferior in any way, is important to the healing process. By being alert to danger signs, the health care professional can be a resource and provide support to depressed or suicidal clients. Listening carefully for any danger signs that the client may be suicidal is critical. An easy mnemonic can be used to remember the warning signs: IS PATH WARM?

I	Ideation	W	Withdrawal
S	Substance abuse	A	Anger
P	Purposelessness	R	Recklessness
A	Anxiety	M	Mood changes
T	Trapped		
H	Hopelessness		

EXERCISES

Exercise 1

Identify your personal responses when feeling "blue" or "down in the dumps." Are these responses healthy or unhealthy? Do they promote resolution to problems or mask and internalize the problem? This exercise is designed for your use only and need not be shared with others.

Exercise 2

Using the Internet, look for self-help bulletin boards or other electronic reference sources that could help you, family members, or clients understand and manage depression. Make a list of the resources found to share with the class.

Exercise 3

Develop a file containing suicide intervention resources for your community. Each resource should include the facility name, address, telephone number, operation hours, specific types of services they offer, fee for services, and any special notes you receive through your interview with the resource.

Exercise 4

Identify the steps you would take if a friend began to send either verbal or nonverbal messages about committing suicide. How would you respond?

Exercise 5

Using the Internet, look for self-help bulletin boards or other electronic reference sources that could help you, family members, or clients understand suicide, those at risk, and intervention approaches. List each resource and summarize pertinent information contained in each site. Begin with the Centers for Disease Control and Prevention site (www.http://cdc.gov).

REVIEW QUESTIONS

Multiple Choice

1. Minor depression is also known as
    a. dysthymia.
    b. reactive depression.
    c. bipolar depression.
    d. endogenous depression.

2. All are true of major depression *except* that
    a. the client may have very little energy.
    b. the client may become quiet and withdrawn.
    c. the client may feel inadequate, worthless, or fearful.
    d. it requires no medical treatment.

3. Reactive depression
    a. comes from within.
    b. is considered the most temporary form of depression.
    c. is also known as melancholia.
    d. is also known as SAD.

4. Clinical depression
    a. is caused by SAD.
    b. is also known as PPD.
    c. is depression severe enough to require treatment.
    d. is caused by BPD.

5. All are true of substance-induced mood disorder *except* that
    a. it may be induced by side effects of common prescription drugs.
    b. it is most common in women after menopause.
    c. it may be caused by a combination of drugs and alcohol.
    d. once the medication is discontinued the depressive symptoms stop.

6. All of the following are true of adult depression *except* that

   a. women are twice as likely as men to experience depression.

   b. many adults feel depression is a personal weakness.

   c. men are more socially conditioned to deny depression.

   d. women are more apt to "act out" their feelings in some type of physical violence.

7. Which is *not* an approach used by suicidal people to communicate their plan?

   a. coded written messages

   b. indirect statements

   c. direct statements

   d. coded verbal messages

8. Therapeutic approaches to suicidal people include all of the following *except*

   a. listening.

   b. acknowledging the reality of their suffering.

   c. avoiding arguments and power struggles.

   d. giving pat answers and advice.

FOR FURTHER CONSIDERATION

1. How would you respond therapeutically to the client experiencing reactive depression?

2. Discuss the impact of depression on each stage of the life cycle. How would you respond therapeutically to each age group?

3. Role-play a suicide scenario, with a classmate going through the four stages of contemplating suicide; use the mnemonic IS PATH WARM.

CASE STUDIES

Case Study 1

For months, Esther, a travel agent, has felt very sad. She feels extremely fatigued and lethargic. She finds it difficult to sleep at night, and her appetite has decreased. Though reading was once a passion of hers, lately she lacks the concentration to even focus on the morning paper. She no longer enjoys activities with her friends and family. She is plagued with feelings of hopelessness; often she struggles to make it out of bed in the morning. She finds herself asking what the point is to her life, and wonders if life is even worth living.

1. Identify the symptoms of depression given in this scenario.

2. If you were Esther's friend, how would you respond therapeutically?

3. Does Esther need treatment for her depression?

Case Study 2

Timmy, a second-grader, wasn't feeling like himself. A month ago his best friend moved to another city, leaving Timmy feeling sad, miserable, and with no one to play with. His mom and dad were worried because he was no longer interested in kite-flying, something he had really enjoyed for a long time. Timmy also tried to make excuses for why he should stay home from school. Sometimes Timmy wouldn't go to sleep at night, and he wasn't interested in eating any of his favorite foods. His parents worried about how sad he always seemed. After a month of worry, his parents decided to take Timmy to a family counselor.

1. Is it possible a second-grader could be experiencing depression?

2. What symptoms did Timmy have that indicate depression?

3. How do you think the counselor will help Timmy?

Please note that because Internet resources are of a time-sensitive nature and URL addresses may change or be deleted, searches should also be conducted by association and/or topic.

ENDNOTES

1. Delate, T., Gelenberg, A. J., Simmons, V. A., & Motheral, B. R., (April 2004). Trends in use of Antidepressants in a National Sample of Commercially Insured Pediatric Patients 1998–2002. *Phychiatric Services, 55*(4).

2. Welter, P. (1990). *How to help a friend*. Wheaton, IL: Tyndale House Publishers.

RESOURCES

http://www.healthyplace.com

http://www.ifishoulddie.co.uk

http://www.outsidein.co.uk

http://www.psychologyinfo.com

http://www.suicidology.org

http://www.upliftprogram.com

Frisch, N. C., & Frisch, L. E. (2006). *Psychiatric mental health nursing* (3rd ed.). Albany, NY: Thomson Delmar Learning.

Lindh, W. Q., Pooler, M. S., Tamparo C. D., & Dahl, B. M. (2006). *Comprehensive medical assisting: administrative and clinical competencies* (3rd ed.). Albany, NY: Thomson Delmar Learning.

Milliken, M. E. (2004). *Understanding human behavior: a guide for health care providers* (6th ed.). Albany, NY: Thomson Delmar Learning.

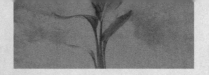

CHAPTER

8

THE THERAPEUTIC RESPONSE TO CLIENTS WITH SUBSTANCE USE DISORDERS

CHAPTER OBJECTIVES

The learner should strive to meet the following chapter objectives and demonstrate an understanding of the facts and principles presented in this chapter through written and oral communication.

- Define key terms as presented in the glossary.

- Compare/contrast substance dependence and substance abuse.

- Describe physiological and psychological dependence upon a drug.

- Discuss whether addiction is a disease or a choice.

- List eight substances commonly abused.

- Identify the reasons clients often give for abusing their substance of choice.

- Compare/contrast the use, misuse, and abuse of drugs.

- Describe important characteristics for addiction treatment.

- Discuss the therapeutic approach to clients who are addicted.

INTRODUCTION

Substance abuse and addiction, referred to as *substance use disorders (SUDs)* continue to be a major health and social problem in our society. SUDs gravely impact the general public, the demands on health care, family dynamics, and the individual.

DIAGNOSIS OF SUBSTANCE USE DISORDERS

Most clients *use* drugs of one kind or another for medical reasons and do so according to instructions. To *misuse* a drug implies that the directions for the drug use are exceeded. The *abuse* of a drug implies that it is used for other than medical purposes. Any drug can be used inappropriately. The lines between use, misuse, and abuse can be easily blurred, causing a problem to surface. Individuals who are dependent upon or abuse substances do so for many reasons, but generally there is a strong need to relieve tension, to relax, to forget about their troubles, and to help them cope with the daily demands of society. In 2001 more than 4.6 million individuals met the DSM-IV criteria for treatment of substance abuse.

The *DSM-IV* is the **Diagnostic and Statistical Manual of Mental Disorders** used by mental health care professionals to promote accurate diagnosis and treatment of mental disorders. There is a criterion for both substance dependence and substance abuse.

Substance Dependence

Substance dependence refers to substance use during a 12-month period that leads to significant impairment, manifested by *three* or more of the following: 1) tolerance; 2) withdrawal; 3) taking the substance in larger amounts over a longer period than intended; 4) desire for the substance is persistent or efforts to control the substance use are unsuccessful; 5) major time is spent in activities to obtain the substance, use the substance, or recover from the effects of the substance; 6) social or occupational activities are diminished because of substance use; and 7) use of the substance continues in spite of persistent or recurrent physical or psychological problems associated with the substance.

Substance Abuse

Substance abuse refers to substance use during a 12-month period that leads to significant impairment manifested by *one* or more of the following: 1) recurrent substance use that results in a failure to fulfill major obligations at work, school, or home; 2) continued use of substance in situations that are physically hazardous to self and others; 3) continued use of substance that creates problems with legal authorities; and 4) continued use of substance in spite of persistent or recurrent physical or psychological problems associated with the substance.

Addiction

Addiction is defined as either physiological or psychological dependence on a substance that is beyond voluntary control. *Physiological* or *physical dependence* implies that the body chemistry has been so affected that withdrawal from the substance produces a physical reaction at the cellular level, sometimes with severe complications. *Psychological dependence* means that the individual craves the substance being abused for the "good feeling" it provides. This need for the substance and the support it gives is viewed as a coping mechanism.

There is an ongoing debate among professionals as to whether addiction is a disease, is a choice, has a genetic and/or developmental basis, or is a combination of each of these. It is not the purpose of this text to bring an end to this debate. While it is likely true that an individual at risk for addiction makes a conscious choice at one point to smoke, drink, or use a drug, there is growing evidence to support the disease factor and/or a genetic/developmental factor in substance use disorders. Accepting drug dependence or abuse as a disease, however, does not totally erase or excuse the responsibility of an addict's actions. This debate will, in part, dictate treatment protocols, also.

A well-known program that shows success with addicted people is Alcoholics Anonymous (AA). AA is a self-help organization for alcohol and substance abusers that is self-supporting and nondenominational. The AA program is based upon following a 12-step program that helps individuals live without their drug of choice. AA sponsors meetings in nearly every community in the country to help addicted people develop a close bond with others with similar problems. AA believes that an addicted person is completely responsible for his/her own recovery. There is a strong religious flavor to AA that some individuals dislike; however, statistics indicate that people following a 12-step program and who are active in AA meetings have a 50 percent greater chance at success in recovery.

COMMONLY ABUSED SUBSTANCES

Some of the more commonly abused substances are identified here, with just a brief overview of their use and effect.

Nicotine is highly addictive in any form. Nicotine or tobacco is smoked or chewed. Even when many cities are banning smoking from all public places, smoking is still seen as the most socially acceptable form of addiction. Some health care professionals would label nicotine addiction as a slow form of suicide. It is a chronic and relapsing addiction that often results in serious illness. Smokers have a risk of cancers of the lungs, mouth, throat, stomach, and bladder, and are prone to cardiovascular disease. Tobacco use in early years may be indicated in later mental illness. The danger of secondhand smoke is also well known. The Centers for Disease Control and Prevention state that tobacco is the single greatest cause of preventable death in the United States. Because nicotine is physiologically addictive, the smoker who quits experiences physical withdrawal symptoms that may include anxiety, agitation, weight gain, and insomnia. It is very difficult to stop using nicotine. Many who are addicted are unable to do so without assistance. Support groups may be helpful; also, there are drugs available to make breaking the addiction and preventing relapse more manageable. They come in the form of prescription gum, patches, and oral medications.

Alcohol, both socially acceptable and legal, also is one of the most commonly abused drugs in society. Alcohol produces a temporary feeling of well-being, but is a depressant that acts upon the central nervous system. Intoxication depends upon the amount of alcohol in the bloodstream, with an amount between 0.08 and 0.10 being considered as legally intoxicated. An intoxicated person suffers slowed thinking and reaction time, impaired vision, poor coordination, and altered judgment as a result of the drug's action. After the initial euphoria and increased motor activity come clumsiness and staggering gait. Nausea and vomiting may occur. Withdrawal symptoms include anxiety, insomnia, tremors, and delirium. Alcoholism is generally identified in three stages—early-, middle-, and late-stage alcoholism.

In the early stage, the occasional drinker begins to drink to avoid problems or to bolster confidence. There is an increase in the individual's ability to tolerate alcohol, and large amounts may be consumed without the individual appearing impaired. In the middle stage, drinking is more intense and begins earlier in the day. The individual is losing control over drinking, usually denies a problem with alcohol, may have blackouts, and begins to suffer serious physical symptoms. In the late stage of alcoholism, the individual is totally obsessed with alcohol, internal organs have been damaged, malnutrition is evident, and death follows if treatment is not received.

Marijuana is a drug under much debate as states consider its legalization. Some believe it is beneficial in reducing nausea and vomiting for those receiving chemotherapy. Others argue that new combinations of chemotherapy drugs reduce nausea and vomiting, making the use of marijuana unnecessary. Marijuana is, however, recognized by the **Drug Enforcement Agency** (see Table 8-1) as a Schedule I drug with little or no benefit and high potential for abuse. Marijuana comes from the dried tops of the cannabis or hemp plant. It has many different street names, including grass, pot, weed, and joint. It is smoked or swallowed. A state of euphoria, altered judgment, and altered perception results from its use. Slowed thinking and reaction time, as well as confusion and impaired balance, are exhibited. A person abusing marijuana may have symptoms of lethargy, hunger, agitation, cough, and frequent respiratory infections. There is a debate among experts as to whether there are withdrawal symptoms from the use of marijuana.

Barbiturates and tranquilizers, found in Schedules II, III, IV, and V, depress the central nervous system, causing symptoms of lethargy and sleepiness. Speech may be slurred, heart rate is slowed, and blood pressure may be lowered. These drugs have significant use therapeutically, but can be highly addictive, leading to both physiological and psychological dependence. These drugs are often prescribed for the

TABLE 8-1   Controlled Substances Act, Federal Drug Enforcement Administration*

SCHEDULE I

- Substance has high potential for abuse.
- No currently accepted medical use in treatment.
- Lack of safety for use of the substance under medical supervision.

Examples include marijuana, heroin, Ecstasy, psilocybin, LSD, peyote.

SCHEDULE II

- Substance has high potential for abuse.
- Has a currently accepted medical use or medical use accepted with severe restrictions.
- Abuse may lead to severe psychological or physical dependence.

Examples include cocaine, Ritalin, opium, oxycodone, morphine, amphetamines, secobarbital

SCHEDULE III

- Substance has less potential for abuse than substances in Schedules I and II.
- Substance has a currently accepted medical use.
- Abuse may lead to moderate or low physical dependence or high psychological dependence.

Examples include anabolic steroids, ketamine, paregoric, hydrocodone, Rohypnol.

SCHEDULE IV

- Substance has a low potential for abuse relative to substances in Schedule III.
- Substance has a currently accepted medical use.
- Abuse may lead to limited physical dependence or psychological dependence relative to substances in Schedule III.

Examples include Valium, Librium, Xanax, Ambien, Darvon.

SCHEDULE V

- Substance has low potential for abuse relative to substances in Schedule IV.
- Substance has a currently accepted medical use.
- Abuse may lead to limited physical dependence or psychological dependence relative to substances in Schedule IV.

Examples include cough suppressants containing small amounts of codeine and preparations containing small amounts of opium.

While the federal law has five schedules, some states have added a Schedule VI to cover substances abused recreationally. They include substances such as those found in spray paints, and nitrous oxide, found in many types of aerosol cans. Because pseudoephedrine is widely used in the manufacture of methamphetamine, some states have strict regulations regarding the sale of any cold remedy containing pseudoephedrine. These drugs include Sudafed and Actifed.

*United States Code of Federal Regulations, Title 21.

treatment of certain stress disorders, for relief of insomnia and pain, and to prevent seizures. Dependence upon these drugs may be so strong that individuals cannot function normally after withdrawal. Valium is one of the most abused drugs in this category. Withdrawal symptoms may not occur until a week or more after discontinuing the drug and may include anxiety, insomnia, and tremors.

Opiates are used medically to control pain. They also can be used to reduce gastrointestinal motility, to curb nausea and vomiting, and to suppress the cough reflex. Opiates come from the opium poppy seed, but are also synthetically made in the laboratory. Heroin, morphine, and codeine are examples of opiates. When abused, stupor, decreased respiration, unconsciousness, and coma can result. Opiates are listed in all five of the Drug Schedule classifications, and are highly addictive when abused. These drugs are generally injected, swallowed, or smoked. Withdrawal symptoms include watery eyes, runny nose, decreased appetite, irritability, tremors, chills and sweats, cramps, and nausea.

Cocaine comes from the coca plant, but can also be manufactured in the laboratory. Cocaine is a strong stimulant to the central nervous system, and is used medically as an anesthetic. In surgery, it can deaden a local area and produce vasoconstriction to reduce bleeding at the site. When abused, cocaine is sniffed or snorted into the nose, rubbed on the mucous membranes, or injected. It creates a euphoria that lasts about 30 minutes, leaving an individual with a greater need each time to have more. It is quick and severe in its addiction and creates multiple side effects that can include cardiac arrhythmias, seizures, respiratory arrest, and death. Crack cocaine is smoked. Withdrawal symptoms include apathy, long periods of sleep, irritability, and depression.

Amphetamines excite the *central nervous system*. Used medically, it can treat short-term fatigue, some respiratory conditions, depression, and narcolepsy. *Methamphetamine* is the most commonly abused drug in this category. It is easily manufactured by anyone having the right ingredients, and is a major concern for law enforcement officials around the country. Methamphetamine gives the user a short-term feeling of exhilaration, energy, and increased mental alertness. Adverse affects include aggression, violence, psychotic behavior, paranoia, hallucinations, cardiac and neurological damage, and impaired memory and learning. Withdrawal symptoms are the same as for cocaine.

Hallucinogens also excite the central nervous system. They have no medical use. These drugs cause hallucinations, mood changes, and delusions. They elevate all vital signs and are highly addicting. Abusers may experience the hallucinations for up to a year following treatment and withdrawal. Most abusers lose touch with reality. They also may injure themselves or others while under the influence. Paranoia, psychosis, and unpleasant "flashbacks" are common. These drugs are usually in the form of lysergic acid diethylamide (LSD), mescaline (peyote), and psilocybin (magic mushroom).

Inhalants—unstable and unpredictable chemical substances in such household items as glue, gasoline, and aerosol spray paints—are often abused by teenagers seeking a "cheap" thrill. They can produce significant behavioral and psychological changes in an individual, such as apathy or aggression and dizziness or slurred speech. The use of inhalants is widespread and dangerous, but often is not classified as addictive because only a small portion of users become dependent. However, abuse of inhalants can lead to coma or, in some cases, even death.

OTHER ADDICTIONS

Health care professionals may become aware of other addictions that can occur in clients' lives. Individuals may become addicted to sexual activity, to gambling, to shopping, to spending hours on the Internet, or to any activity that gives a high-adrenaline rush to the pleasure center of their brains. Some authorities believe chronic overeating may constitute a substance abuse disorder and should be considered an addiction. The Centers for Disease Control and Prevention (CDC) report that more than half of all the adults in the United States are overweight. Obesity increases the risk of cardiovascular disease, stroke, diabetes, and hypertension. As food becomes more palatable, more pleasurable, and more refined, it also is consumed in much larger quantities than necessary. When food becomes an addiction, it is being consumed not to satisfy a normal hunger, but to achieve a pleasurable reward, no matter what the consequences.

TREATMENT

Primary care health care professionals who are alert and diligent about getting a thorough social history from clients may uncover a tendency upon the part of clients to drink too much or to rely upon drugs to cope with daily living. Because many health problems are associated with substance dependence and abuse, health care professionals may be the first to diagnose a substance dependence or abuse problem.

STOP AND CONSIDER

You are a medical assistant interviewing Jana, the expectant mother identified in the opening case study. You are asking her the questions on the social history form. She tells you she does not smoke. She does not drink coffee, but she drinks cola products nearly every day. In response to the questions on alcohol, she is a little evasive. Since Jana volunteered to you earlier that she is fearful she might be an alcoholic, you know the goal is for her to be truthful to you now.

1. What might you say to open the communication?
2. What questions will you ask?

Mental health care professionals working in concert with primary care health care professionals also often reveal substance dependence and/or abuse. The first step is to recognize the problem; the second step is proper treatment. Most treatment plans will include a number of days of **detoxification** as an inpatient in a treatment facility, to begin to rid the body of the abused substance. This period may include the administration of medications. Following detoxification, treatment must continue with close and careful monitoring, counseling, and support to enable individuals to remain free of substance abuse. Studies show the following factors are significant in the worsening health of individuals addicted to a substance: female gender, living alone, problem use of opiates and/or alcohol, having no medical insurance, older age, and clients who abuse more than one substance. When the brain has been affected by the abuse of substances, many individuals turn to risky sexual behaviors, thus increasing their health risk for transmission of infectious diseases, including HIV.

A client needing treatment feels caught in a vicious cycle that begins with excessive use of a drug: disapproval—self-recrimination—guilt—rationalization and denial (defense mechanisms)—continued excessive use of a drug (see Figure 8-1). One of the keys to successful treatment is to break this cycle so the client can move toward recovery. Appropriate treatment will likely be different for each client, but the following points are important:

- No single treatment will work for everyone.
- Treatment should be readily available, even without medical insurance.
- Medical detoxification is only the beginning of treatment for long-term drug use.
- An adequate period of time is necessary for treatment effectiveness.
- Individual and/or group counseling is critical to treatment.

- Treatment should tend to *all* the needs of the individual, including medical services, family therapy, vocational rehabilitation, and social and legal services as necessary.

- Medications are increasingly successful in assisting the treatment process.

- Treatment for drug addiction is a long-term process and often requires multiple episodes of treatment.

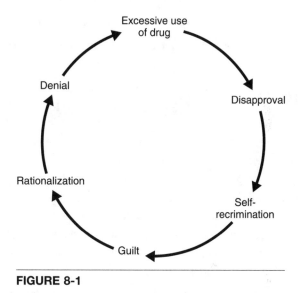

FIGURE 8-1

The Role of Family and Friends in Drug Dependency

It is important to briefly discuss the role of family members and friends in the treatment of drug dependency. The disease is a problem that affects the entire family. Everyone near the addict suffers. It is not possible or beneficial to try to cajole, beg, or intimidate the drug-dependent person into changing. Persons with substance use disorders can only decide for themselves to give up the drugs they abuse. Family members may even become part of the problem when they try to conceal their loved one's addiction. This is done by making excuses to employers, giving money when they should not, and generally enabling the drug-dependent person to remain dependent, thereby not facing up to the reality of the problem. There are many support groups dealing with the problem of codependency and numerous books written on the subject.

Health professionals must also be careful not to become codependent to the problem.

There are five Cs to recall when working with substance-dependent clients. They were identified many years ago, and have been useful to many who live or work with drug dependency.

Remember:

- I did not CAUSE the disease.

- I cannot CURE the disease.

- I cannot CONTROL the disease or the substance-dependent client.

- And if I try to, I CONTRIBUTE to the problem, and I go CRAZY.

THE THERAPEUTIC RESPONSE

Health care professionals may have more difficulty maintaining a therapeutic relationship with addicted clients than with clients seeking other kind of medical care because the chance for relapse is so great. It can be depressing to watch a client slip back into destructive habits after many months, even years of being free from the abuse. Health care professionals must strive for an unbiased approach to their clients and see their role as one of helping clients choose recovery. Collaboration will be expected from all professionals caring for the person with an addiction problem. The following points can help health care professionals be more therapeutic in their approach:

- Become educated regarding substance dependency and abuse. You cannot be therapeutic toward a problem you do not understand.

- Identify people at risk in your client population. These can include, but are not limited to, children of drug dependents, people with high-stress lives, individuals who have easy access to substances, individuals with unresolved emotional problems, and individuals with chronic and debilitating health issues.

- Encourage clients to seek treatment when there is a problem. Help them understand the available resources and make referrals as appropriate.

- Do not moralize or scold clients for their behavior. Everyone else does that to them.

- Manage any negative feelings you have.

- Do not be discouraged, and do not believe you can "fix it."

- Elicit the cooperation and participation of family members and friends in the treatment process. Help them understand the codependency cycle.

- Be tolerant of clients who relapse. Be willing to start again with clients who fail or drop out of treatment.

continues

The Therapeutic Response continued

- Attitudes of compassion, understanding, patience, and acceptance are the best therapeutic approaches to drug dependent clients. Such a relationship fosters positive motivation for the client who needs strong support in their recovery process.

SUMMARY

It is rare today to find a family that is not touched in one way or another by the problem of substance use disorders. It is a major problem for society as a whole, as well as for all of health care. Health care professionals will be able to respond more therapeutically if they are well informed and stay up to date on the latest developments for substance dependence and abuse. It is important to understand the culture of the community in which you are employed, to be nonjudgmental in your approach to drug-dependent clients, and to provide as much support as possible. Have a ready list of available resources and services for clients and their families. A partial list of national resources is provided for you here:

- Alcoholics Anonymous: www.aa.org
- Drug Abuse Resistance Education: www.dare.com
- MedlinePlus (Substance Abuse Problems/Topics): www.nlm.nih.gov/medlineplus/substanceabuseproblems.html
- National Institute on Drug Abuse: www.nida.nih.gov
- Substance Abuse and Mental Health Services Administration (SAMHSA): www.samhsa.gov

EXERCISES

Exercise 1

If you live in an area large enough to have a treatment center for individuals who abuse drugs, interview the administrator or a counselor. If you are in an area that does not have any treatment facilities, search using the Internet for treatment centers. Your goals are to discover the following:

1. What resources are available in the community?
2. What are the most commonly abused substances they see in their clients?
3. What factors make their treatment successful?

4. What problems are faced by clients when discharged?

5. What is the cost of treatment, and who pays if there is no health insurance?

6. How are families involved, if they are at all, in the treatment plan?

Write a summary of the information you received and describe what you learned from the experience.

Exercise 2

Using the Internet, research Alcoholics Anonymous to determine their 12-step program approach. Would these 12 steps work for individuals from all cultures? Justify your response.

Exercise 3

A client says to you, "I need to go outside to have a smoke while I wait for the doctor."

You feel_____.

You respond_____.

A client says to you, "Can the doctor help me stop smoking?"

You feel_____.

You respond_____.

A client says to you, "My pain medication is no longer working so good. Can you make sure I get something stronger from the doc?"

You feel_____.

You respond_____.

A veteran from the war in Afghanistan comes to your clinic for his second round of drug abuse treatment.

You feel_____.

You respond_____.

Exercise 4

Write a brief paragraph about someone you know who abuses a substance. What is your response to that individual? Are you codependent? Why or why not? Describe any action you might be able to take to help that individual.

REVIEW QUESTIONS

Multiple Choice

1. The most commonly abused substance in the U.S. is
   - **a.** alcohol.
   - **b.** prescriptive drugs.
   - **c.** nicotine.
   - **d.** methamphetamine.

2. The standard tool used by mental health care professionals to promote accurate diagnosis and treatment of mental disorders is called the
   - **a.** ICD10-CM.
   - **b.** SUD.
   - **c.** CPT.
   - **d.** DSM-IV.

3. When the body chemistry is so affected that withdrawal from the substance produces a reaction at the cellular level, sometimes with severe complications, the terms is
   - **a.** physiological dependence.
   - **b.** psychological dependence.
   - **c.** chemical dependence.
   - **d.** chemical abuse.

4. A drug that may be abused, is currently listed as a Schedule I drug, but is being legalized in a number of states is
   - **a.** cocaine.
   - **b.** marijuana.
   - **c.** Valium.
   - **d.** heroin.

5. Barbiturates and tranquilizers
   - **a.** stimulate the central nervous system.
   - **b.** cause lethargy and sleepiness.
   - **c.** depress the central nervous system.
   - **d.** both b and c above.

6. LSD is a/an
   - **a.** amphetamine.
   - **b.** opiate.
   - **c.** tranquilizer.
   - **d.** hallucinogen.

7. Addiction is likely
   - **a.** a choice.
   - **b.** a disease.
   - **c.** related to genetics and development.
   - **d.** a combination of all the above.

FOR FURTHER CONSIDERATION

1. You have just heard your 16-year-old daughter return home from a date. She is getting ready for bed. You step into her room to ask her how the date was and to kiss her good night. You are immediately overwhelmed by the smell of pot. What do you say? What will you do? Where might you go for resources?

2. The school board in your community has voted to randomly test for drugs all students who participate in extracurricular activities. Your son, a better-than-average football player, says he'll not play another day on the team if he has to pee in a cup for anyone! What is your response? Can you identify both positive and negative aspects of the school board's decision?

CASE STUDIES

Case Study 1

Your physician employer has asked you to put together some information for Jana, the client identified at the beginning of this chapter who is pregnant with her first child and believes she has an alcohol problem. What information will you include? What resources will you recommend to her? Identify any community resources available. Provide information about her health needs and the health needs of her unborn infant during pregnancy.

Case Study 2

Roxann Piersen is a long-term client in your ambulatory care medical center who suffers from severe headaches and debilitating back pain. You have reason to believe she is abusing her pain medications. Your chart notes indicate that either she or her pharmacy calls for refills on her prescription prior to the time when she should be out of her medications. You have two notes, one indicating she accidentally spilled most of her pills down the sink, and another note saying she lost the medications on a vacation. What action do you take? Explain.

RESOURCES

American Psychiatric Association (2000). *Diagnostic and statistical manual of mental disorders* (4th ed.). Washington, DC: American Psychiatric Association.

Frisch, N. C., & Frisch, L. E. (2006). *Psychiatric mental health nursing* (3rd ed.). Clifton Park, NY: Thomson Delmar Learning.

The National Institute on Drug Abuse. www.nida.nih.gov.

The Substance Abuse and Mental Health Services Administration (SAM HSA). www.samhsa.gov.

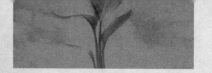

CHAPTER
9

THE THERAPEUTIC RESPONSE TO CLIENTS WITH LIFE-ALTERING ILLNESS

CHAPTER OBJECTIVES

The learner should strive to meet the following chapter objectives and demonstrate an understanding of the facts and principles presented in this chapter through written and oral communication.

- Define key terms as presented in the glossary.
- Compare/contrast acute illness, chronic illness, and life-altering illness.
- Identify typical phases of life-altering illness clients may experience.
- Differentiate between curative care and palliative care.
- Describe several psychological effects of illness.
- Discuss the use of medications and life-altering illness.
- Discuss cultural influences on life-altering illness.
- Identify appropriate therapeutic responses to chronic and life-altering illness.

OPENING CASE STUDY

I was 25 years of age, and my daughter was just 7 months old, when I learned that a tumor on the right lobe of my thyroid gland had to be removed. Surgical procedures went well, and the doctor felt everything would be all right. Four days later my physician came to the hospital room and asked if I would walk down to the sunroom with him. We sat down; he pulled his chair close to mine and took hold of my hand. "Billie, there is no easy way to tell you this, but your lab results came back positive for cancer. We must do radical surgery to remove the remainder of the thyroid and to see how far the cancer has spread." As his words began to sink in, he added, "I want you to call your husband. When he arrives, I will come back in to speak with him, too."

The next few days were rather like a blur. The surgery was scheduled. Arrangements were made with a friend to take care of my daughter. My sister would come from Texas to help after surgery. At that time, the only treatment for cancer of this type was radical surgery. Because the doctor was not sure if or how far the cancer might have metastasized, and the cervical region has an abundance of lymph nodes, the surgery would be extensive. An incision was made from my right ear along the jaw line to the center of my chin. Another incision was made down the side of my neck and to my mid-thoracic region. A third incision was made around the front of my neck and out to the end of my right shoulder. I think of it now as being like a side of beef hung out to cure before being cut into serving portions. Or as my friend said, like a "live autopsy."

For three days after surgery in the hospital, I knew nothing. When I was lucid, the surgeon told me that he took two of my parathyroid glands as well as the thyroid. He told me I would need to take medicine the rest of my life—but he had saved my life. I was grateful. I also did not fully understand what would happen next. When I came home, I could not climb the few stairs to the bedroom, so I slept on the couch. The pain was so bad, however, that I could not stand to have anything touch me; I could not wear my clothes. My sister touched me lightly with *a cotton ball, and I screamed with pain. I awoke one night with my body on fire. I could see a fire in the fireplace and I screamed for my husband. "I am on fire!" He said, "No, you're not." But I could feel my skin burning; I just couldn't smell the burned flesh. When I called the physician the next day, his response was "Thank God. That burning sensation means your nerves are regenerating." (Too bad he hadn't told me to expect this.)*

For one entire year, I could not function without assistance. My sister stayed with me six weeks after the surgery, then friends and neighbors helped as much as possible. It was next to impossible to raise my right arm, to wash or comb my hair; even to dress myself was a chore. I could not pick up my daughter. She had to be put on my lap for me to hold and love. The teenagers from the church where my husband and I were youth advisors got off the school bus near our house every day after school. They helped with my daughter, rinsed the soiled diapers (there were no disposables or diaper services then), did my wash, cleaned the house, and got dinner started before they left for home.

During this time, I learned that my other two parathyroid glands had atrophied from the trauma of surgery and were no longer functioning. Now I had no thyroid gland to secrete the thyroid hormones tetraiodothyronine (thyroxine or T4) and triiodothyronine (T3)—the hormones essential for life that have many effects on body metabolism, growth, and development. I also had no parathyroid glands to secrete parathyroid hormone (PTH) necessary to regulate the amount of calcium in my blood. Calcium is a critical element for the nervous system, the muscular system, and the skeletal system. When calcium levels drop below normal (which mine certainly had by now), tingling sensations in the fingers and/or cramps in the muscles of the hands are common. When the calcium level is too low, I feel foggy, strange, or like my brain isn't working quite right.

Gradually, my life began to return to normal, although the struggles were sometimes unbearable. I was able to take care of myself, be the kind of mother I wanted to be, and go on with my life. I was able to have another child; our son was born five years after my surgery. The physician had warned us that to have a child any earlier could be dangerous because of the increased hormone activity during pregnancy. I now thought I was home free; however, I still panicked each year when it was time for my annual physical examination. Would the cancer return?

Living with thyroid replacement medication is not too difficult, and keeping the replacement hormone at just the right level has been fairly simple. Regulating the calcium level in the blood is quite a different story. I faithfully took the medicine; I took five Ultra Tums three times a day plus 1.25mg of Vitamin D four times a week. Most people do not require extra doses of Vitamin D because so many of our foods are fortified with it today. After 20 years on this regime, everything began to go wrong.

I began to lose my appetite and then became extremely nauseous. The nausea became so severe I could not keep water or even ice chips down. I lost 20 pounds. My doctor did not know what was happening, and I felt like he thought I was just making up my symptoms. He thought a scan might tell him something. When I got no relief, and began to run a fever because I was so dehydrated, I called the doctor again. I told him I was on my way to the emergency room. If he wanted to meet me there, it was okay; otherwise I was going to seek out another physician. My doctor met me at the emergency room. By now he knew my symptoms were not all "in my head." He called for an internist. Blood tests were run, and both my calcium levels and blood pressure were sky-high. Because Vitamin D is stored in the body (primarily in the kidneys), taking too much over a period of time can cause poisoning and even death; my body had reached a dangerously high level. I spent a week in the hospital being pumped with IV fluids to flush out my system. It was discovered that some permanent damage had taken place in my kidneys.

After 42 years, I am still learning to live with this life-altering illness and continue to be treated by the same internist. I know that if my Vitamin D level drops too low or is all used up, I get tetany; my body becomes one giant charley horse. Every muscle hurts: the large leg muscles, the muscles in my feet and hands, even the little tiny muscles around the eyes. I know what it is like to receive calcium IV, because for six months, three times a week, I received calcium this way. It feels like rivers of molten lava as it moves through the blood vessels; I get red and flushed, and feel like I am on fire again. I also know what to expect if my Vitamin D level is too high; my blood pressure climbs to a dangerous level, and nausea and vomiting ensue. I watch my activity level and the amount of exercise I do each day. I know when to take extra calcium. I have some shoulder limitations. I cannot bowl, or pitch horseshoes, and I must be careful lifting. Any tension seems to move to the smaller shoulder muscles, which spasm and twitch. I have iatrogenic Horner's Syndrome, causing problems with my right pupil dilating, ptosis of the right eyelid and loss of sweating over the right side of my face. When I am over-heated, half my face is white and dry while the other half is beet-red and sweaty.

I live a rich and full life in spite of these problems. I am about the best grandma around, I help sail our 34-foot sailboat with my husband, and we travel and have seen beautiful places around the world. I went back to school, earned my medical assisting degree, worked in a medical clinic, and later became my former instructor's assistant in the medical assisting program at a community college. My supervisor suggested to me one day that I might like to teach. I thought she was crazy; the only teaching I had ever done was with 2-year-olds in Sunday school. I tried it; I really liked it. I went back to school and earned my vocational teaching certification. When my supervisor moved into another position, I began to teach full-time. Later, I rewrote the curriculum into self-paced modules with open enrollment, in order to offer all students an opportunity for education. I am a co-author of this text and of a major medical assistant text.

I decided long ago that my attitude was critical to my well-being. I accepted my illness. I choose to live life to the fullest. I maintain a positive attitude, look for the good in everyone and everything, and encourage others. I am more sympathetic to individuals who have health issues because of my life experience. My hope is that everyone might experience a primary care physician who listens, respects the issues they have, provides honest feedback, and genuinely cares about the uniqueness of each person.

—Billie Lindh

INTRODUCTION

As illness progresses from a minor inconvenience to the impending death of the client, the aspects of therapeutic communication change. Health care professionals spend most of their time in diagnosing and educating clients in the care of acute illness. As illness progresses to a life-altering stage, the health care professional must shift emphasis toward emotional, cultural, financial, and legal issues in meeting the clients' needs. Meeting this need in a therapeutic manner becomes challenging.

ILLNESS TYPES

Most illnesses are unexpected and always bring daily and/or life changes. There seems to be no good time for illness. Illnesses come in many different forms, some lasting only hours and others impacting lives in significant ways. Illnesses can be characterized as **acute**, **chronic**, and **life-altering**. The majority of acute illnesses do not progress into the chronic or terminal phase. A chronic illness, however, may become life-altering.

Acute Illness

Clients with *acute illness* experience a rapid onset of the illness with severe symptoms, most often for a short duration. These clients may not be able to perform the tasks of daily living and may be unable to continue their occupational employment until the illness has run its course. Acute illnesses can be classified as an inconvenience, and do not normally result in life changes. Examples of acute illnesses include a cold, the flu, tonsillitis, or rashes. Left untreated, acute illnesses may progress into chronic conditions. Symptoms of acute illnesses may include fever, diarrhea, nausea, vomiting, stomach cramps, and inflammation. Medical personnel need to help the client understand any implications of the diagnosis and assist them in making decisions regarding their medical care.

Chronic Illness

An illness is usually labeled *chronic* when its symptoms linger over a period of time. While some chronic illnesses may be cured within a few weeks or months, many may last a lifetime. Chronic illnesses typically have a significant impact on clients, necessitating life-altering changes as they attempt to cope with the illness, comply with treatments, and deal with possible side effects. The illness may gradually debilitate and shorten their life spans. At some point, an illness that shortens an individual's life span may become life-threatening.

It is not the purpose of this text to identify specific diseases and clients' possible reactions to them, but the following examples of illnesses may be particularly challenging over a long period of time:

- Arthritis
- Fibromyalgia
- Multiple Sclerosis
- Type I Diabetes Mellitus
- Diabetic neuropathy
- Cancer
- Acquired Immunodeficiency Syndrome (AIDS)
- Emphysema
- Chronic Obstructive Pulmonary Disease (COPD)
- End-stage renal disease

Communicating therapeutically with individuals with chronic illness requires an extra dose of the characteristics identified in Chapter 3, The Helping Interview.

Personalities and life experiences are extremely varied, but it is likely that clients with serious chronic illness will experience the same stages of grief identified for those who grieve the loss of a loved one—denial, anger, bargaining, depression, and acceptance. (See section in Chapter 10.) It is also likely that these clients may never get to the stage of acceptance, because it is so easy to become mired in the other stages. When health care professionals know what stage of grief a client is in, especially when the client is first diagnosed, they can better understand and respond therapeutically. If clients learn to accept their illness, they may quickly return to another stage when another health crisis occurs, either with their existing illness or with a new illness. It can be a vicious cycle, giving clients burdens they may or may not be able to handle. Remember, too, that their family members may go through the stages of grief as well, but be in different stages at different times than the clients, complicating communication and interactions.

It cannot be said strongly enough that a health care professional will need to express warmth and caring, be genuine and honest with clients, listen and function with a sympathetic and empathetic ear, and assist clients in living their lives to the fullest. None of this can be accomplished unless a health care professional is comfortable with chronically ill individuals and is nonjudgmental in all aspects of care. Referring clients and their family members to illness-specific support groups such as the American Cancer Society and the Arthritis Foundation provides education opportunities, emotional support, and others who know firsthand just what is being experienced. Medical social workers are also available to educate, instruct, and support clients and their families.

Life-Altering Illness

When chronic illness progresses to the stage when death is the inevitable result, the illness is defined as *life-threatening*; however, some chronic illnesses and most life-threatening illnesses are categorized as life-altering illnesses. A life-altering diagnosis creates feelings of powerlessness and lack of control. Hope should always be maintained, however, as in some cases the disease may be fought for years before ultimately ending in death. Therapeutic responses should emphasize the positive.

Clients with life-altering illnesses may try to convince themselves that nothing is wrong or deny the diagnosis. For some, this period provides time to come to terms with what is happening and to cope with the range of emotions they feel. As the diagnosis is processed and accepted, feelings of anger may be hurled toward the physician, health care professionals, or family members and friends. "How could you let this happen? I've been coming in for my annual physical exam. Why didn't you tell me about the risks?" Many clients fear the symptoms of the illness and pain, but not death itself. Once the client reaches the acceptance stage of their prognosis, they worry about what will happen to their spouse, partner, and family, especially children, once they are gone. The health care professional should not attempt to direct the client to make final decisions—updating a will or signing a physicians' directive or durable power of attorney for health care—until they have reached the acceptance stage.

Clients in the final stages of a life-threatening illness may find that medical goals change from curing an illness or prolonging life to providing comfort, focusing on **palliative** care. Palliative care provides relief from the client's physical symptoms such as pain, shortness of breath, and nausea, as well as satisfying emotional needs and helping with stress management for the client and family members. Sometimes this care is provided in a **hospice** environment. The philosophy of hospice affirms life, regards dying as a normal process, and neither hastens nor postpones death. Hospice clients have made a decision to spend their last days at home or in a homelike setting. Hospice provides personalized services and a caring community so that clients and families can attend to the preparations for death that are satisfactory to them. Professional medical care is given and symptom relief provided. The client and the family are both included in the care plan, and emotional, spiritual, and practical support is given based on the client's wishes and the family's needs.

LOSSES FACED BY INDIVIDUALS WITH A LIFE-ALTERING ILLNESS

Persons who are chronically ill, persons who face a life-altering illness, and persons who are dying suffer great losses. They grieve their loss of good health, their independence, their body image, their lifestyle, and their sense of self-confidence (see Figure 9-1). If they need constant medical care and attention, they may grieve their loss of privacy and modesty. Their daily routine is interrupted. Their financial security is usually threatened.

Relationships change. Some are lost; new ones are made. Established work and home roles are radically altered and daily routine is different. Plans for the future may be dashed. It may be impossible to participate in leisure activities once greatly enjoyed.

Sexual functioning may be altered. Health care professionals are equipped to discuss this alteration, but sadly it is not always done, because either the client or the health care professional feels uncomfortable in doing so. What is and is not possible with a disability should be discussed. What other forms of sexual expression might be encouraged if sexual intercourse is impossible is a question that needs to be addressed.

It is important to keep persons who suffer from a chronic or life-altering illness or who are dying as comfortable as possible. Attend to their physical needs, teach them how to safely monitor their medications, provide them as much control as possible, answer their questions honestly, and also remember the concerns of family members. Embrace their culture as much as possible.

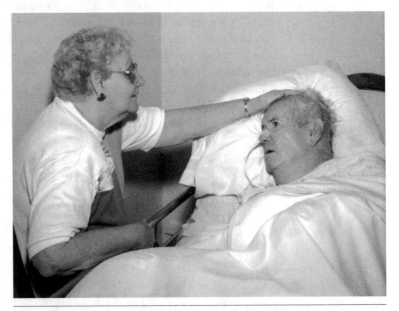

FIGURE 9-1

STOP AND CONSIDER

1. What therapeutic actions do you see demonstrated in the opening case study?
2. What other therapeutic responses might you have used if you were caring for Billie in the hospital?
3. Where would you put Billie on Maslow's Hierarchy of Needs during the various phases of her life-altering illness?

PSYCHOLOGICAL EFFECT OF LIFE-ALTERING ILLNESS

The basic personality of clients with life-altering illnesses may be changed significantly, depending on their psychological experiences. For example, the client who has always been thoughtful and kind may suddenly speak harshly or swear at those providing care. Or someone who is normally calm and loving may have periods of violence and hostility. Some clients who seem happy and upbeat most of the time may slump into a deep depression.

Personal relationships may also change during a life-altering illness. Your best friend may not be able to cope with watching you suffer, and may find excuses not to visit in order to manage their own guilt feelings. Some cope with their discomfort with terminally ill clients by rushing around doing whatever, just to keep busy. The client might prefer to simply have company, someone to just sit with them, to hold their hand, to listen. For some, it is difficult to touch or caress a dying person. The dying person may be the one to reject any close contact or relationships as well.

Setting personal goals for the client faced with a life-altering illness is an activity that distracts their focus away from the primary illness and toward therapeutic activities. Examples of personal goals may include the following:

- Establish goals to achieve something each week. This might include calling a friend to chat, taking a short walk, or writing a letter to a friend.

- Plan some things to look forward to in the long- as well as the short-term. Seeing a daughter married may be a short-term goal; seeing a grandchild born may be a long-term goal.

- Sign a physicians' directive or living will, and a Durable Power of Attorney for Health Care.

- Update the last will and testament and arrange financial and personal affairs.

- Discuss any worries about pain and symptom control with medical professionals at an early stage.

- Learn about the illness and what to expect.

It is important to project a tolerant attitude toward family decisions such as withholding medications or heroic measures to preserve life. An intolerant attitude by medical personnel, at this time that is so stressful for both client and family members, is emotionally disturbing. Health care professionals must be available to respond to questions; to listen; to be nonjudgmental when choices are made that might be different from their own; and to be considerate, respectful, and polite at all times.

MEDICATION CONSIDERATIONS

Whether the client chooses hospitalization or hospice care, medications will be involved. These medications may include analgesics for pain, sedatives for sleep, medications to treat the specific disease, antidepressants, tranquilizers, the administration of oxygen, and the list goes on. Health care personnel have been educated as to how and when to administer medications and understand the risks and side effects involved. When the responsibility of administering medications is delegated to a family member, the situation can be problematic. The client or family member may feel the dosage is too strong and not give the prescribed amount. Or they may feel their loved one will become addicted to the medication if a large dose is given or if it is given too often. Many do not understand that it is important to take pain medication as it is prescribed, whether or not the client is in pain when the medication is due. Waiting too long to take the medication only renders it ineffective and causes unnecessary discomfort for the client. It is important for health care professionals to communicate to caregivers the need to strictly adhere to medical directions regarding medication.

CULTURAL INFLUENCES ON LIFE-ALTERING ILLNESS

Modern technology has made it possible to live longer and to remain in a terminal stage longer. Because of technology, the end of life may have more difficulties for the client and family members. The following are considerations that need to be addressed in order to avoid end-of-life difficulties.

- Has a living will or physicians' directive been signed?

- Has a Durable Power of Attorney for Health Care been established?

- What cultural values and beliefs should be considered?

The following are just a few of the cultural influences to be considered. Should the client be told he or she has a life-altering illness? For most Americans, the answer would be yes; it is one of the basic patient rights to know. Other cultures, however, may value the family over the individual. For example, studies reveal that over half of the Mexican-American population feels that dying clients should not be told their prognosis. This is also true of many Korean Americans. In Asian countries, such as China and Japan, it is customary for the physician to reveal the diagnosis only to the client's family. It is up to the family whether or not to tell the client.

Some cultures consider it insensitive to tell a client he or she is dying. They feel it creates a sense of hopelessness and actually may hasten the dying process. Other cultures feel that the stress of knowing the condition would only cause the condition to worsen. Still others believe that only God knows when someone will die. The Hmong believe that to tell someone they are dying is to curse them. They wonder how you could know they would die unless you plan to kill them yourself?

It is important to remember that not all members of the same culture will make the same choices. For example, two Filipino families experienced the death of a family member. One of the families followed the traditional pattern of withholding the life-threatening diagnosis from the client. After the death, the family was pleased with their decision, as their loved one was able to live out her days without the added burden of knowing she was dying. The other family decided to tell the client the diagnosis. After the death, they felt satisfied with their decision, knowing that their loved one was able to make her final arrangements and say good-bye to family members. As health care professionals, we must be careful not to impose American values on others, and not to stereotype cultures.

THE THERAPEUTIC RESPONSE

- Understand the importance of cultural values and beliefs and do not stereotype.
- Be prepared for mood swings and realize that these may be part of the process of coming to terms with what is happening.
- Encourage open and honest discussion about emotions and feelings. Sometimes just listening and understanding demonstrates a therapeutic response.
- Include the client and family in discussions about a treatment plan.
- Allow the client to make decisions whenever possible.
- Discuss any worries the client may have about pain or symptom control and their management.
- Educate family members about the illness and what to expect.
- Help the client and family members manage their stress.
- Deal with the present, the here and now.

SUMMARY

All illness is, at best, an inconvenience. However, when the illness becomes chronic or life-altering, serious decisions must be made. Health care professionals will be called upon to help educate the client about the illness, what to expect, treatment regimens, and prognosis. It will be important for health care professionals to consider cultural differences when providing information and to not allow their personal biases and prejudices to hinder the therapeutic response. Expressing warmth and caring, being genuine and honest, listening, and assisting clients in living their lives to the fullest are appropriate therapeutic responses. Providing community resources is also helpful for the client and family members.

EXERCISES

Exercise 1

Determine what support groups are available in your community for persons with AIDS. Select a group, make a phone call to a representative of the group, and discuss how you might volunteer your assistance.

Exercise 2

Using the Internet and your favorite search engine, look for information about three cultural values and beliefs, different from your own, regarding life-threatening illness, prolonging life, and rituals associated with death and burial. Compile this information to be shared and discussed with classmates.

Exercise 3

Using the Internet and your favorite search engine, look for information about hospice care in or near your community.

- What are the client qualifications for hospice care?

- Collect as much information as you can and compile it in a notebook.

- Are there other resources for the client experiencing life-altering illnesses in or near your community?

REVIEW QUESTIONS

Multiple Choice

1. Acute illness
   - **a.** lingers over a period of time.
   - **b.** includes an experience of some stages of grief by the client.
   - **c.** includes diseases such as COPD, cancer, and AIDS.
   - **d.** has a rapid onset with severe symptoms and a short duration.

2. Palliative care involves all of the following *except*

   a. curing the illness and prolonging life.

   b. providing relief from physical symptoms.

   c. providing relief from emotional symptoms.

   d. helping with anxiety and stress management for the client and the family.

3. _____ affirms life, regards dying as a normal process, and neither hastens nor postpones death.

   a. Terminal illness

   b. Chronic illness

   c. Hospice

   d. Acute illness

4. All of the following are true of the psychological effect of illness *except* that

   a. the client may experience basic personality changes.

   b. the client who is normally thoughtful and kind may speak harshly.

   c. the client who normally is calm and loving may become violent.

   d. the happy client may slump into deep depression.

5. Therapeutic responses to the client experiencing life-altering illness include all of the following *except*

   a. encouraging open and honest discussion about feelings.

   b. understanding the importance of cultural values and beliefs.

   c. stereotyping, which is always effective when considering cultural values and beliefs.

   d. helping the client and family members manage their stress.

FOR FURTHER CONSIDERATION

1. How do different types of illness (acute, chronic, and life-altering) impact the client and family members?

2. If you were diagnosed today with a life-altering illness, how would you feel and respond?

3. Do you feel there should be a different approach to medications for the client experiencing a chronic illness and the client whose death is imminent?

Case Studies

Case Study 1

Suzanne, a hospice nurse, was assigned to manage the home care of Maria, a Spanish-speaking Mexican woman with metastatic breast cancer. Maria was receiving both chemotherapy and radiation; however, the cancer was progressing rapidly. Family members were close and loving and translated for Maria and Suzanne. Maria was desperately fighting not to let her disease upset normal family routines.

After two weeks of managing the case, Suzanne sensed an underlying strain. She felt the family was not coping as well as outward appearances indicated. Maria was choosing to compromise her comfort in order to maintain her traditional role in the family as wife and mother. She was becoming increasingly exhausted and withdrawn.

Suzanne decided to call in a bilingual/bicultural colleague to help assess the problem. Maria was able to talk more openly to the colleague when family members did not have to translate everything for Suzanne. Translating through her family members meant that Maria could not be as open and honest, because she had to pretend she was doing well and maintaining normalcy.

1. Using the Internet, research the Mexican culture's views on family values and beliefs, and how these might impact life-threatening illnesses.

2. How would your rate Suzanne's evaluation of this situation?

Case Study 2

An elderly Iranian woman was slowly dying. The hospital staff felt that nothing could be done to improve her condition. Her son refused to sign the Do Not Resuscitate (DNR) order and insisted that everything possible be done to prolong his mother's life. Staff members could not understand this reasoning, and felt that it was causing needless suffering for the client.

1. Using the Internet, research the Iranian culture's family values and beliefs, and how these might impact life-altering and life-threatening illnesses.

2. Why is it important to understand other cultures' values and beliefs associated with health care issues?

3. How are cultural situations handled when the views of health care professionals and clients are different?

RESOURCES

Lewis, M. A., & Tamparo, C. D. (2002). *Medical law ethics & bioethics for ambulatory care* (5th ed.). Philadelphia, PA: F. A. Davis Company.

Lindh, W. Q., Pooler, M. S., Tamparo, C. D., & Dahl, B. M. (2006). *Comprehensive medical assisting: administrative and clinical competencies* (3rd ed.). Albany, NY: Thomson Delmar Learning.

Luckmann, J. (2000). *Transcultural communication in health care.* Albany, NY: Thomson Delmar Learning.

Milliken, M. E., & Honeycutt, A. (2004). *Understanding human behavior: a guide for health care providers* (7th ed.). Albany, NY: Thomson Delmar Learning.

Purnell, L. D., & Paulanka, B. J. (2003). *Transcultural health care a culturally competent approach* (2nd ed.). Philadelphia, PA: F. A. Davis Company.

Tamparo, C. D., & Lewis, M. A. (2005). *Diseases of the human body* (4th ed.). Philadelphia, PA: F. A. Davis Company.

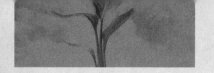

CHAPTER

10

THE THERAPEUTIC RESPONSE TO CLIENTS EXPERIENCING LOSS, GRIEF, DYING, AND DEATH

CHAPTER OBJECTIVES

The learner should strive to meet the following chapter objectives and demonstrate an understanding of the facts and principles presented in this chapter through written and oral communication.

- Define key terms as presented in the glossary.

- Describe Dr. George L. Engel's three processes for working through grief.

- Discuss Dr. Elisabeth Kübler-Ross's five stages of grief and dying.

- Identify at least six cultural differences in grief and death experiences.

- Identify five kinds of losses.

- Describe how age factors can influence grief.

- Compare/contrast how men and women express grief.

- Explain the difficulties family members have in the grieving process.

- Define anticipatory grief.

- Define dysfunctional and unresolved grief.

- Compare/contrast life-threatening illnesses versus terminal illnesses.

- List at least seven therapeutic responses to grief and death.

- Discuss the impact a physicians' directive has on dying and death.
- Discuss recent legislation in the right-to-die issue.

OPENING CASE STUDY

Bob felt a sharp and piercing pain in his head, his eyes blurred, and he passed out. Later, after many tests, he learned that he had a benign but inoperable tumor that had spread like a spiderweb through his brain. Family and friends rallied to help with Bob's care. Treatment began, in the hope of shrinking the tumor.

The night of his death, only a few months later, he told his wife, "I'm going to beat this. I know it is going to be gone when I have my next brain scan." Bob never moved from the denial stage throughout his short illness.

INTRODUCTION

Grief, dying, and death are very personal. Dying is a process. Death is an event. Grief is a response. Everyone has experienced grief from the loss of someone or something that had great meaning. Many, if not all, have experienced the death of a significant person in their lives. Others may be suffering from a life-threatening illness.

To be therapeutic with people grieving and dying implies, at least in part, coming to terms with one's own death. This can be accomplished by gaining knowledge and experience in the grieving and dying process.

GEORGE L. ENGEL, M.D., 1913–1999

George L. Engel, M.D., was a distinguished physician and teacher who devoted much of his career to investigating human relationships in the context of health, death, and loss. He identified three processes or stages of working through grief. They are 1) experiencing disbelief or shock over the loss, 2) realizing that the loss did occur, and 3) acknowledging the loss in a realistic manner.

During the shock and disbelief process, individuals may withdraw from social interaction or have difficulty carrying out normal daily activities. They may also have physical symptoms of sighing, shortness of breath, lack of appetite, and inability to sleep. When individuals are finally beginning to realize the loss in the second process, feelings of guilt, anger, and frustration are common. Accepting the loss is the time when individuals have a desire to renew their lives and look to the future. They are able to face the loss in a realistic manner.

DR. ELISABETH KÜBLER-ROSS, 1926–2004

Another classic theory comes from Elisabeth Kübler-Ross in her book *On Death and Dying. In the book, she presents five stages people may experience upon learning they are dying. In the years since 1969, and with much referral to these stages by health care professionals and others, the stages are now known as the "five stages of grief and loss."*

1. *Denial*: This is the time when people deny reality.

2. *Anger*: This is the time when people express their anger and rage.

3. *Bargaining*: This is the time when people are willing to do anything to change what has or is happening to them. ("Let my son live, and I'll become a better person.")

4. *Depression*: Expect deep sorrow and feelings of aloneness when the loss is recognized.

5. *Acceptance*: This is the realistic acknowledgment of the loss.

Kübler-Ross also learned from her research that there was no order to the stages and that some people never make it through all the stages. In reality, these stages are now applied to all types of grief and loss. The research also recognized that individuals might pass through all the stages several times in doing their grief work.

CULTURAL INFLUENCES ON GRIEF AND DEATH

A person's culture and heritage have a significant influence on the manner in which grief and death are met. Consider some of the following questions and examples for a better understanding of culture's role.

Do you place flowers on a grave for the dead person to smell, or do you place tools and food in a grave for the dead person's journey? Does your culture view death as a process the entire family embraces, or is grief an emotion to be borne alone? Would you and your family be most comfortable if you died in the hospital or in familiar surroundings at home? Is the hospital viewed as a place of death or a place for care and treatment?

In some cultures, end-of-life decisions are seldom made by the client, making hospital requirements that every person be asked about end-of-life choices upon admission difficult to achieve. Family members or the eldest child (in some cultures, the eldest son) may step in and make the decision, with the client's permission. Many prefer to die at home because of the belief that dying elsewhere means their soul will wander around with no place to rest. It is not permissible to discuss serious illness or death in some cultures. Some prohibit autopsy unless required by law and view organ donation as body mutilation.

The death ritual may be many different events. For some, it is a celebration of life; for others, the funeral is a social event that involves a long service, the body on display, and burial with a favorite possession. For others, it is a time of deep sorrow and weeping. Some families will delay the death ritual so that friends and family can travel long distances to arrive for the event. Others must bury their dead within 24 to 48 hours. In the Islamic faith, the dead person will be washed three times by someone of the same sex and wrapped in white material prior to a prompt burial. In some cultures, it is appropriate to wear black as a sign of mourning; in others, white is worn. Some cultures will have family, friends, and loved ones keep watch around the clock over individuals who are dying or who have died; the idea is to never leave this person alone. Some release balloons at a grave; others sprinkle rice wine around the grave. Some family members in mourning cover mirrors in their homes to decrease focus on appearance; others wear black arm bands or white head bands. Some cultures bring gifts of money as well as food for the bereaved; others send sympathy cards.

Some cultures remember the dead on the anniversary of their death. Failure to do so would rob the living of rest. Some individuals return to gravesites yearly to clean the grave of weeds and debris, talk with the deceased, and share a picnic with family and friends. Others never return to the gravesite. Some are cremated, with ashes spread at sea or in a favorite place.

Health care professionals unaware of cultural differences may find themselves in uncomfortable situations, or feel embarrassed by saying or doing something that is inappropriate. It is important to obtain as much transcultural information as possible in order to respond and communicate in a therapeutic manner.

KINDS OF LOSSES

World events afford everyone an opportunity to discover the kind of grief that accompanies loss. Devastating weather events like hurricane Katrina, which left so many homeless; the Indonesian tsunami that destroyed homes and lives; and drought and fires that burn farmland, forests, and residences provide ample opportunity to understand the kind of grief that comes from loss. Also, daily reports from war-ravaged countries show the loss of lives and the suffering of survivors. The many children in Africa who are left without parents because so many lives have been lost to AIDS provide another example of the loss of loved ones. Pick up any newspaper; listen to any radio or television broadcast; grief and loss will be reported.

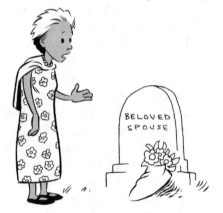

"I'VE HAD SO MANY
LOSSES LATELY."

Health care professionals will find that there are several kinds of losses that cause grief. They include 1) the loss of personal possessions that have a great deal of meaning, such as a home destroyed by fire; 2) the loss of a familiar environment, such as a person experiences who must move from an area especially enjoyed or who loses his/her job; 3) the loss of a significant other in a person's life—life partner, parent, child, close friend, family pet, etc.; 4) the loss of some part of self—for example, the loss of a limb, the loss of hearing or sight, or even the loss of psychological function such as memory, self-confidence, or respect and love; and finally,

5) the loss of life itself. In the loss of life, the concern is usually not so much from the death itself as it is from the fear of pain and the loss of control over one's life. For some, death is seen as a release or an entry into another life; for others, death and its separation and abandonment are seen as something to fear.

✤ CASE STUDY ✤

Juliene was going to visit her 85-year-old mother in an assisted living apartment. It soon would be Christmas. She had with her a table-size decorated tree and a small nativity scene. She also had a small plate of the kind of fudge they made together during the holidays. Christmas was an important time for both of them; there were so many memories of decorating the Christmas tree and putting out the nativity. Juliene's mother was suffering from Alzheimer's disease and had been failing rapidly. When Juliene arrived, her mother seemed pleased to see her, immediately ate a piece of fudge, but ignored the Christmas tree and the nativity scene. Juliene put the tree on the table and placed the nativity underneath it, chatting all the while. Her mother seemed confused. Finally, she was able to say, pointing to the tree, "What is that?" As Juliene explained, it was clear that her mother did not understand. Juliene's eyes filled with tears as she realized she had lost another part of her mother. She cried all the way home.

FACTORS THAT INFLUENCE GRIEF

A person's age will, in part, determine how one reacts to grief. *Infants* know only that there is a loss if someone is not there to feed, clothe, hold, and love them. *Toddlers* are confused and cannot distinguish animate from inanimate. Does the chair cry when it is broken? They feel anxious if someone is not there to care for them. *Children aged 3 to 5 years* believe that death is reversible. They think the dead person may just be sleeping; they are curious about life and death. *Children aged 6 to 10 years* are very curious about death. Is it cold in the ground? Can the dead move? What happens to the body? They want to do their own funeral ritual. This age group may dig up a dead pet to see what has happened to it. They may feel very guilty about a divorce, blaming themselves and feeling like Mom and Dad do not love them anymore. *Adolescents* have a fascination and a fear about death. They repress and deny feelings and do not talk about a loss in peer groups unless it is the death of one of their own; then they dwell on it. As common as divorce is in our society, adolescents still are devastated by divorce. Adolescents may need help from an older person they care about to cope with their grief. *Adults* sense that loss poses a threat to their pattern of living, perhaps their financial status, but are beginning to examine their own life and its meaning. *Older adults* grieve the aging process, grieve for their friends who have died, and fear a loss of independence.

Men usually have a more difficult time expressing grief openly, since they are mostly expected by society to be strong and supportive. *Women* generally have an easier time expressing grief, since they are perceived as needing the support of others. The opposite may be closer to the truth. It is fairly common in a retirement community for a man to follow his wife in death by only a few months, while a woman may pick up, change her life, and live many years after her husband has died. This may be in part because, traditionally, women throughout their lives are more likely to have a support network of friends to help them deal with their loss. A man more often than not sees his life partner as the person with whom he can talk and share grief. When that person is no longer present, it is difficult to grieve alone.

It has been said that the greatest grief comes from the loss of a child. Even if a person is 80 years of age and loses a child aged 60, the loss is as great as the loss of a young child. The loss of an unborn infant falls in this category, also.

Everyone grieves at a different rate and in different stages. That is why it is so difficult for family members to help one another. One person may be in denial while the other is in depression; one is angry while the other is in acceptance. It is easy to "blame" the other person for no help or support. It is usually impossible for spouses and partners to help each other in any way other than to share their love and their sadness. For this reason, it can be important to seek outside help in their grieving process.

Anticipatory Grief

Anticipatory grief occurs when individuals do part of the grieving process prior to the actual loss. People with life-threatening illnesses, people who are dying, and people who know they are going to lose a part of themselves begin the grief process early. This can be beneficial, if it helps individuals progress to a healthier state after the loss has occurred. It is not beneficial if individuals dwell upon the anticipated loss for extended periods. The most difficult grief work usually occurs when the relationship has been one with a fair amount of conflict, ambivalence, and unspoken messages. It is better to spend some time clearing up unfinished business and stating important messages to those close to you before a loss occurs. Many times grief is heightened by the fact that harsh words were spoken during the last encounter prior to death. Anticipatory grief simplifies the grieving process later.

STOP AND CONSIDER

Recall the case study where Juliene is visiting her ill mother before Christmas.

1. What kind of grief is Juliene experiencing? Explain.
2. Is her mother grieving? Why or why not?
3. What can be done to help Juliene through this process?

Dysfunctional and Unresolved Grief

Since everyone grieves at his/her own pace, and because there is really no one "right" way to grieve, caution must be used in labeling **dysfunctional** or **unresolved grief**. There are a few considerations to keep in mind, however, that may be helpful. Dysfunctional and unresolved grief can cause unexplained somatic responses, some stress-related medical diseases, and altered relationships with friends and relatives. An inability to cope with loss is disruptive to a person's physiological and psychological functioning. This process may be characterized by uncontrolled crying, hopelessness, helplessness, intense reactions lasting longer than six months, alterations in eating and sleep patterns, denial of loss, idealization of the lost person or object, and a constant reliving of past experiences.

Another kind of unresolved grief may be more difficult to resolve. This kind of grief comes when there is no finish or completion to the death event. A good example is the grief experienced by family members of individuals missing in action (MIAs). These people may know only that a body was not found and that their loved one is presumed dead. Crime victims whose bodies are never recovered, victims who are lost at sea—these, too, are examples of death that does not have a final event.

It is often beneficial for grieving family members to establish some kind of completion process. This might include a legal pronouncement of death, observing a death ritual, or planting a tree in the name of the person who is gone. Even pronouncing that the grief has ended and life is beginning again can be helpful.

Losses Faced by Individuals with a Life-Threatening Illness

The term *life-threatening* is used in this text as opposed to *terminal*. The reason should be obvious, but the use of *life-threatening* rather than *terminal* allows a place for hope and empowers a person to a higher degree of control over the circumstances. Individuals who receive the news that their illness is life-threatening realize that death may be imminent. This knowledge is different from the news that an illness is life-altering, since life-threatening implies that there may be only a little time left. When an individual who has been cancer-free for more than five years discovers the cancer has returned and is raging through several vital organs, there is a real threat to survival. There is no reprieve.

If clients are not in denial about a life-threatening illness, they may come to feel that there is an advantage in knowing that death is imminent. Individuals are more likely to make preparations for their final days. Are there people to say good-bye to? Do they need to seek forgiveness or forgive someone? Are financial matters in order? Are end-of-life decisions in place? Do they have any regrets? Is there anything they want to do, someplace they want to go, someone they wish to speak to? If there is a project that needs to be finished, they may hasten to complete it. Some will tell friends and family of their diagnosis and that they do not have much time left. Others prefer that no one know the seriousness of their illness, so that no one will treat them differently. Some who know they are dying choose to do nothing differently because they try to live each day as if it might be their last. Others are glad to know that life is shortened, because it allows them to put in place some action they had not taken the time to do previously. They find a new joy in life and may regret that they did not make the best of every day they had. One thing is fairly certain, however: grieving will occur.

THE RIGHT TO DIE

No matter in what context grief, dying, and death are discussed today, the topic of a person's right to die will likely surface. Advance directives and federal legislation in the Patient Self-Determination Act require health care institutions that receive Medicare and Medicaid reimbursement to establish written policies and procedures on advance directives, allowing individuals the right to identify clear choices in their death. At the risk of being too simplistic, there are at least two reasons why the courts and individual state constitutions have passed legislation on this issue.

The first reason is that physicians are taught to preserve life. Death may be seen as failure. Allowing individuals to die, even when there is no hope for survival, is very difficult, even impossible for some. The second reason is that technology looks at death as another fatal disease to conquer at all costs. Medical technology has advanced much faster than has ethics. Without warning, dying individuals often get caught in a system in which technology has ultimate control.

One thing is certainly a result of all the publicity and discussion over an individual's right to die with dignity, to ask that no heroic measures be used, and to even seek assistance with death: individuals may be better informed and may have made decisions about their death prior to facing the event. These decisions may be reduced to writing in a legal document called a living will or a physicians' directive.

Medical office personnel may receive such directives from those individuals whom their physicians treat. The directives should be discussed with their physicians and filed in their charts. When a person is hospitalized, a copy of the directive should be sent to the hospital. While the client's wishes should be respected and followed, health care professionals cannot be expected to act unethically or illegally. Any problems should be openly discussed to resolution.

Dying individuals and family members may request that attending physicians keep the dying comfortable and free from pain. Some people who know they are dying may ask physicians if they can be given an injection or receive medication to end their life. The latter is more likely to occur when the dying process is slow, painful, debilitating, and likely to render a person unconscious. While refusing to commit an illegal act, physicians can be therapeutic at such a time by acknowledging and accepting the desperation felt, discussing with their clients how their pain can be managed, and assuring family members that suffering can be kept to a minimum.

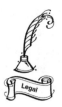

Helping others to die is both a controversy and a debate in this country. Often the debate is fueled by those who have watched loved ones suffer immeasurably in their dying. Oregon was the first state to pass an assisted death law. Voters approved the law twice, but it was faced with a great deal of conflict both in and out of the court system. Finally, the U.S. Supreme Court ruled against John Ashcroft, the U.S. Attorney at the time, to protect, by ballot, Oregon's right to choose assisted death. While the numbers in Oregon who use the law each year are small, many of the state's residents find comfort and hope from the control that has been given to them. Aid in dying legislation is pending in a number of states. The controversy grows, however, and with it comes the possibility of opposing legislation referred to as "health decision restrictions" that would make it difficult to withdraw nutrition and/or hydration from a permanently unconscious person. Legislation of this type is filled with emotion and faces both legal and ethical challenges on both sides of the issue.

Assisted suicide is the term used when someone provides the means for a person to end his or her life. *Euthanasia* is the term used when someone intentionally acts to terminate the life of a suffering individual. The Netherlands is the only country that allows both. Interestingly enough, individuals discussing their death choices while well and healthy will often propose such measures; however, the closer one is to death, the greater is the desire to delegate such decision-making to professionals. As medical technology and science advance, the problem of how and when to prolong life will become more complex.

It may be helpful to remember that technology is a tool that does not have to be used. Life is not an idol to be worshipped. There is a time to die. Caring may very well be more important than curing.

In his book *Anatomy of an Illness,* Norman Cousins made this statement:

"Death is not the ultimate tragedy of life. The ultimate tragedy is depersonalization—dying in an alien and sterile area, separated from spiritual nourishment that comes from being able to reach out to a loving hand, separated from desire to experience the things that make life worth living, separated from hope."

THE THERAPEUTIC RESPONSE

Responding therapeutically to individuals who are grieving a loss or facing death is a challenge. Recall the suggestions made in Chapter 9 related to the loss and grief that accompanies a life-altering illness. Generally, health care professionals are advised to keep their emotions distant from those they serve. The distance protects them from experiencing the same loss as their clients face. Such a distance cannot always be maintained, however, and perhaps it should not be. Medical providers who are too professional, appear aloof, or do not experience their clients' loss and grief serve only a part of their clients' needs. Recognizing the stages that clients might be experiencing and responding appropriately will go a long way to facilitate therapeutic communication. For instance, clients in the anger stage of loss may vent their anger toward you. Remember that their true anger is for the loss; it is not personal, toward you. Keep in mind the following:

- Accept individuals where they are and in what they are experiencing.

- Acknowledge individual cultural beliefs and values expressed during grief.

- Listen to what is being said; listen to what is not being said.

- You cannot move a person out of denial. You can only help the person remain as close to reality as possible.

- Do not take any expressed anger personally. Be aware that you may try to avoid individuals who are angry. Avoidance is a roadblock to communication.

- Do not be embarrassed by clients' emotions or your emotions.

- Do not give false assurances or avoid discussing any problems that may be uncomfortable but must be addressed.

- Refer clients to counselors, clergy, attorneys, social workers, and/or hospice as appropriate.

- Answer clients' questions honestly and simply; they may forget your responses and ask again.

- Put information in writing for clients to refer to at a later time.

continues

The Therapeutic Response continued

- Words may not be necessary, but if they are, it is most appropriate to say, "I am sorry. What can I do to help?"

- Honor clients' wishes with respect, even if they do not agree with your beliefs.

- Enable the dying person to remain independent as long as possible.

- Provide clients as much dignity as possible.

- Recognize that life-threatening illnesses take a great deal of energy. Help the individual conserve energy as much as possible.

- Demonstrate compassion and understanding.

- As a health care professional, do not view death as a failure of your profession. It is a part of the continuum of life.

- Allow yourself a "breather"—a time to draw away from the intensity of grief.

- Take care of yourself so you can take care of your clients.

- Leave the grief you experience in your professional setting where it is; do not take it home with you.

SUMMARY

Recall the stages or processes that individuals who are grieving are likely to experience. Respect the many cultural variances surrounding grief and death. If you are uncertain about what rituals are appropriate, ask your clients. They will be relieved to tell you their wishes. Learn to recognize what might be dysfunctional or unresolved grief and seek ways to assist clients through the process. Understand the legal guidelines in the state in which you are employed related to issues surrounding death and the observance of living wills, physicians' directives, and clients' wishes.

Because health care professionals care for the sick and those who are facing death, they are likely to experience grief from the loss of a client or experience the grief expressed by clients because of some serious loss in their lives. Being present with these clients, listening to their grief, remembering that they are fragile at this time, and providing support and assistance as appropriate are the most therapeutic responses you can give.

On a personal note, it has been said that until you suffer a great loss, you cannot fully understand the depths of the sorrow and suffering that is called grief. If you have experienced heartbreaking loss, you are a part of the brotherhood and sisterhood of those who have felt the searing heat from the fire of deep sorrow. When you understand such loss, you know that suffering rips you open, but you also know that into that space flows compassion, if you will let it in.

In this process, take care of yourself and remember that you cannot be of help to others unless you are in touch with your own emotions. Seek advice and comfort from those around you, and allow time to process and recover from the loss. If you are employed in an environment where death occurs fairly frequently (long-term care facilities, oncology, or hospice), recognize that release from the stress caused by the loss is essential.

Finally, there is no need to ask yourself if you are strong enough to cope; you will be if you believe you can be. Strength comes from within. Remember the butterfly that comes wet-winged from its own chrysalis: from darkness into light; from confinement into freedom.

EXERCISES

Exercise 1

With a friend or classmate, discuss what kinds of choices you would make if you knew you were dying. What kind of medical care would you select? What would be most important to you? Write a brief report identifying your choices.

Exercise 2

Plan your funeral, memorial service, or death ritual. Discuss your choices with family members. Write a brief report describing your service.

Read the obituaries in the local newspaper. Then draft your own as you might see it in the newspaper.

REVIEW QUESTIONS

Multiple Choice

1. Which of the following statements is correct?

   a. Grief is an event, dying is a process, death is a response.

   b. Dying is a process, death is an event, grief is a response.

   c. Dying is an event, death is a process, grief is a response.

   d. Dying is a process, death is a response, grief is an event.

2. George L. Engel, M.D., identified

   a. five stages of grief.

   b. three stages of grief.

   c. three processes of working through grief.

   d. five processes of working through grief.

3. In death rituals,
   a. flowers are always present.
   b. gifts of money and food are unwelcome.
   c. black is the most appropriate color worn.
   d. culture will determine the protocol.

4. It is believed that the greatest loss is
   a. the death of a child.
   b. the death of a spouse or significant other.
   c. the loss of an arm, leg, or eye.
   d. the loss of health.

5. Which of the following is not true?
   a. A person's age will, in part, determine how one reacts to grief.
   b. Children aged 6 to 10 are not curious about death.
   c. Adolescents have a fascination and a fear of death.
   d. Older adults grieve the aging process and fear a loss of independence.

6. Anticipatory grief
   a. occurs when there is no completion to the death event.
   b. is the result of a loss of a loved one who was a crime victim.
   c. means that individuals do part of the grieving prior to the actual loss.
   d. only exists when experiencing a life-threatening illness.

FOR FURTHER CONSIDERATION

1. In the opening case study at the beginning of this chapter, what problems might Bob's family experience because he never moved from the denial stage of his illness?

2. If you were a close relative of Bob's, what would you hope for?

3. It has been said that an individual who is dying and remains in denial never loses hope. Discuss.

4. Do you have a living will or a physician's directive? Why or why not? If not, who would make life-and-death decisions for you if you were unable to?

CASE STUDIES

Case Study 1

Jill Dawson was the mother of a beautiful young woman, Amy, who went to work for a social agency in South America after her college graduation. She loved working with the children in the little village where she and three others had been assigned. After a year in South America, one of the men assigned to the same village made sexual advances to Amy, but Amy was not interested. She tried to be diplomatic in her refusal of his advances. It did not work, however. She reported her discomfort to agency headquarters and asked for a transfer. Their response was to tell her to "work it out."

One month later, the natives heard screams coming from Amy's hut. As they arrived at her door, they saw Jon Peters running out. He dropped a butcher knife as he rode away on his bicycle. Amy was inside with 14 knife wounds in her body. She died before they could get her to medical help. Jill received the dreaded call from the agency, which also informed her that Amy's assailant, one of the other agency employees, had been arrested for the crime. The murder trial was held in South America. Jon Peters was represented by the agency's lawyers, and was found innocent by reason of insanity. He was released into the custody of U.S. officials who accompanied him to the United States, where he was to be held in a mental institution.

Jill grieved for months. She grieved every birthday Amy might have had, she grieved the grandchildren she would never have, and she grieved the loss of a daughter. But, even through that grief, there was consolation in knowing that her murderer would not harm anyone any more.

Twenty years later, Jill was approached by a writer who wanted to tell the story of what had happened to Amy. She agreed to be interviewed. The writer was sensitive and shared information with Jill. While she relived some of the horror, it helped her put into perspective what had happened. She found peace in telling her side of the story. Before the book was published, the writer visited her again. He said, "I don't want you to read this in my book; I must tell you myself. I found Jon Peters. He is living in Ottawa and works as an accountant for the federal government. He is married and has one daughter. He refused my interview requests. My research indicates no criminal record."

1. What can you learn from this story about grief? Does grief ever end? Why or why not?

2. Identify what Jill might have felt after learning the whereabouts of Amy's murderer?

3. If you were Jill, what might help you bring closure to your grief?

Case Study 2

Conner Leonard worked for Purges Manufacturing for 32 years. Along with four other men, he helped to start the company that designed and built products sold around the world. Purges Manufacturing grew and did very well, so well in fact, that other companies wanted to buy it out. The company was sold three times in 12 years. Each time, Conner held on to his job. He was no longer helping in the design process, and had a more difficult time feeling pride in all the parts now made in Mexico. Another buyout was looming. Conner knew he might be outsourced.

1. What kind of grief is Conner feeling? Justify your response.

2. During his annual physical examination, what discussions might occur related to Conner's work?

3. Can you describe what it might be like to say good-bye to a job you loved, to a company you helped to build?

RESOURCES

American Bar Association. www.abanet.org

Anderson, K. (2006, September/October). Katrina meditations. *Spirituality & Health.*

Compassion and Choices. http://www.compassionandchoices.org

EMedicineHealth. Grief and Bereavement. http://www.emedicinehealth.com/grief_and_bereavement/article_em.htm

Holbrook, M., & Tucker, K. (2005, Summer). Improving laws. *Compassion and Choices*, 4(2).

Kiesling, S. (2006, September/October). Wired for compassion. *Spirituality & Health.*

Lewis, M. A., & Tamparo, C. D. (2002). *Medical law, ethics, and bioethics for ambulatory care* (5th ed.). Philadelphia PA: F.A. Davis Company.

Purnell, L. D., & Paulanka, B. J. (2003). *Transcultural health care* (2nd ed.). Philadelphia, PA: F.A. Davis Company.

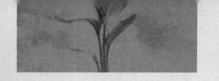

APPENDIX

A

THEORIES OF HUMAN GROWTH AND DEVELOPMENT

INTRODUCTION

The following theoretical views introduce the medical health care professional to human growth and development. The theorists agree that personality and **cognitive** skills build upon each other as physical growth and maturity progress throughout the life cycle. The theories focus on different aspects of development; however, each of the theorists proposes progression through the stages in a sequential manner. This is not an exhaustive listing of developmental theorists, but will provide basic concepts and theories that represent major theorists in this area of study.

To appropriately care for clients, health care professionals must have knowledge of normal behavior for specific age groups and be able to interact on the client's level of understanding. The health care professional may also be involved in teaching primary caregivers how to help their clients through a particular crisis or stage of life.

OVERVIEW OF IVAN PAVLOV AND B. F. SKINNER'S BEHAVIORAL LEARNING THEORIES

Learning theorists recognize that laws of behavior can be applied at any age. Learning theory explores the relationship between stimulus and response. If a hand is waved in your face, the response is automatic—you blink. If you panic each time you pass the corner where you were in a serious accident, the response is learned.

Life is a continuing process of learning. One part of this learning is known as conditioning. Conditioning means that a particular stimulus or experience triggers a particular response.

Two theorists, Ivan Pavlov and B. F. Skinner, described how conditioning is critical to development. The two types of conditioning described are **classical** and **operant**. A brief discussion of these conditioned responses is helpful in further understanding therapeutic communication.

Ivan Pavlov, Behaviorist

Ivan Pavlov (1849–1936), a Russian scientist, is well known for his identification of the earliest and simplest form of learning. He identified **classical conditioning** in his famous dog experiment, which illustrates his theory. Pavlov knew that a dog salivated automatically as a reflex when there is food in its mouth. He presented food to the dog along with the ringing of a loud bell. Eventually the bell alone caused the dog to salivate—the learned response. To further illustrate, study the following example of classical conditioning.

Example of Classical Conditioning

Unconditioned stimulus	=	**Unconditioned response**
—food		—salivation
Conditioning	=	**Unconditioned response**
—food and bell		—salivation
Conditioned stimulus	=	**Conditioned response**
—bell		—salivation

Health care professionals often experience this classical conditioning, as seen in the small child who immediately begins to cry in fear when the assistant enters with a needle. The pain of the needle has been associated with the assistant so often that the child begins to cry just at the sight of the assistant. You may be able to relate similar responses. Some children become quite anxious at the smell they associate with the dental office. Others are afraid when they see someone in a white uniform.

Health care professionals remembering this conditioned response will consider various methods to help alleviate this fear and anxiety. Employees in a pediatric office might wear colors instead of white, or even consider uniforms with children's figures on them. Making the experience as positive as possible will help. The physician might carry a toy or an object of distraction. He/she is advised to spend some time with a child in a nonthreatening manner. The physical setting should include objects that delight a child. Many find a built-in aquarium beneficial. Others use appropriate children's media.

Even adults have conditioned responses that should be considered. A well-known cancer specialist, David Bressler, M.D., purchases juggling bags for his cancer clients. His primary goal is to make certain his clients have something other than the cancer, the pain, and the difficult treatment to associate with him. This physician teaches the client something new about juggling on each visit. They often juggle their bags together. Of course, the added benefits are the laughter and the concentration on the juggling, which take the client's mind off the disease.

B. F. Skinner, Behaviorist

B. F. Skinner (1904–1990) formulated the learning model knows as **operant conditioning**. Skinner and Pavlov agreed that classical conditioning explains some types of behavior. Skinner, however, believed that operant conditioning plays a much more important role.

The difference between classical conditioning and operant conditioning is that in operant conditioning, the response *precedes* the reward. For example, a rat pushes a lever and is rewarded with food. The food is pleasurable and useful, so the rat pushes the lever again. If the reward or consequence of pushing the lever is unpleasant, the rat will not repeat the behavior. Because a person's behavior is what brings the reward, this kind of conditioning may also be called **instrumental conditioning**.

Skinner believed that successful child rearing was accomplished through consistent rewarding of desirable behavior. If the behavior is followed by a pleasant reward or stimulus, the reinforcement is *positive*. If the behavior is followed by the removal of an unpleasant stimulus, the reinforcement is *negative*. Skinner believed that reinforcement was most effective if it was intermittent. Behavior would be rewarded most of the time, but not every time.

There are both *positive* and *negative reinforcements*. A positive reinforcement is something good or pleasant. A negative reinforcement is taking away the bad or unpleasant stimulus. Negative reinforcement is not to be confused with punishment. *Punishment* is an unpleasant event that makes behavior less likely to be repeated.

Remembering this theory is helpful in therapeutic communication. The little girl who is upset and crying because of the injection receives a badge of courage from the assistant for the injection site. As the child is being told how brave she was, and the badge is put on, she begins to feel better and a smile creeps across her face. This is an example of negative reinforcement.

The father who rewards his son with an ice-cream soda because he did such a good job raking the lawn, or the piano teacher who puts a gold star on the piece of music that was memorized are examples of positive reinforcement.

The reinforcement can be primary or secondary. A primary reinforcement is one that is basic and immediately satisfying, such as food. The reinforcement is secondary if the reward itself allows us to get something we want. An example of this is the allowance used as a reward that allows the child to go to the movies with a friend.

It is also helpful to distinguish between negative reinforcement and punishment. In punishment, an unpleasant stimulus is applied to discourage behavior. Punishment may be necessary, but the child can also learn to avoid punishment without changing behavior. For example, a student who receives a failing grade on an exam may avoid the circumstances and skip class rather than fail again. Such behavior requires attention from anyone who has control over the circumstances. The teacher must award the grade earned by the student, but should try to create a positive and encouraging atmosphere for the student, so they will study harder for the next test.

Overview of Sigmund Freud's Psychosexual Stages of Development

Sigmund Freud (1856–1939), a Viennese physician, theorized that all human behavior is energized by *psychodynamic* forces, which he divided into three components. He called these forces the **id**, the **ego**, and the **superego**. In the mentally healthy person, these three forces work together cooperatively and enable the individual to realize fulfillment of basic needs and desires. When the three forces are at odds with one another, individuals are said to be maladjusted. His theory focused on *psychosexual development*, and emphasized that each stage must be conquered before progressing to the next stage.

The Id

Freud identified the id as a person's basic animal nature. It is primarily unconscious and is amoral. It is not governed by laws of reason or logic, and possesses no values or ethics. The id's primary function is to decrease pain and increase pleasure—also known as the **pleasure principle**.

In its earliest form, the id is a reflex response. For example, when a bright light falls on the retina of the eye, the eyelid closes and light is prevented from reaching the retina. The excitations produced in the nervous system by the light can then quiet down to maintain **homeostasis**.

An example of an internal reflex occurs during urination, when a valve in the bladder opens as the pressure on it reaches a certain intensity. The excitation or tension produced by the pressure ends as the contents of the bladder are emptied.

The id retains its infantile character throughout life. It cannot tolerate tension. It wants immediate gratification. It is demanding, impulsive, irrational, selfish, and pleasure-loving. It is the spoiled child personality. The pursuit of pleasure and the avoidance of pain are the only functions that count. It does not think; it only wishes or acts.

The Ego

The ego is the psychological force that is in touch with reality and mediates between the id and the superego. It deals with the outside world in a conscious fashion. The ego is governed by the **reality principle**, *reality* meaning that which exists. The goal of the reality principle is to postpone the discharge of energy until the actual object that will satisfy the need has been discovered or produced. For instance, we must learn to delay gratification (for example, eating when we are hungry, sleeping when we are tired, and so on) until the timing or the situation is appropriate for fulfillment of our needs. This delay of action means that the ego has to be able to tolerate tension until it can be discharged in an appropriate form of behavior.

The institution of the reality principle does not mean that the pleasure principle is forsaken. It is only temporarily suspended. Eventually, the reality principle leads to pleasure, although a person may have to endure some discomfort while looking for reality.

The ego's lines of development are laid down by heredity and guided by natural growth processes. This means that every person has inborn potential for thinking and reasoning that come through experience, training, and education.

The Superego

The **superego** is the moral branch of the personality and represents the ideal rather than the real. It strives for perfection rather than reality or pleasure. The superego is the person's moral code. It develops out of the ego as a consequence of the child's assimilation of his or her parents' or primary caregivers' standards regarding what is good and virtuous and what is bad and sinful.

The superego is made up of two groups, the **ego-ideal** and the **conscience**. The *ego-ideal* corresponds to the child's conceptions of what his or her parents or primary caregivers consider to be morally good. These standards of virtue are conveyed to children by rewards given for conduct that is in line with those standards. If they are consistently rewarded for being neat and tidy, then neatness is apt to become one of their ideals.

Conscience, on the other hand, corresponds to the child's conception of what his or her parents or primary caregivers feel is morally bad, as established through experiences with punishment. If children have been frequently punished for getting dirty, then dirtiness is considered to be something bad.

Freud's Erogenous Zones

Some regions of the body are more likely to experience tensions that can be relieved by some action upon the region, such as sucking or stroking. These areas are referred to as **erogenous zones**. Manipulation of an erogenous zone is satisfying because it affords relief from irritation (such as scratching relieves an itching sensation) and because it induces a pleasurable, sensual feeling.

The principal erogenous zones are the mouth, the anus, and the genital organs. Each of the principal zones is associated with the satisfaction of a vital need: the mouth with eating, the anus with elimination, and the sex organs with reproduction. Freud maintained that the erogenous zones are of great importance for the development of personality, since they are the first sources of tension the infant has to contend with, and they yield the first important experiences of pleasure.

The crux of Freud's theory is that each individual must successfully resolve the needs and conflicts of each stage in order to pass into the succeeding stage. The problem, however, according to Freud, is that many people do not reach the fulfillment of the genital stage and may fall prey to a variety of emotional symptoms and personality problems.

This table illustrates each of Freud's psychosexual stages.

TABLE 1 Freud's Stages of Psychosexual Development

Psychosexual Stage and Age Range	Erogenous Zone	Sexual Activity
Oral (birth to 1 year)	Mouth, lips, tongue,	Sucking, swallowing, chewing, biting, vocalizing
Anal (1 to 3 years)	Anus, buttocks	Expulsion and retention of waste products, toilet training
Phallic (**Oedipus**) (3 to 6 years)	Genitals	Recognize differences between sexes and become curious
Latent (7 to 11 years)	Genitals	Physical and psychic energy are channeled into the acquisition of knowledge and vigorous play
Genital (12 years and older)	Genitals	Puberty and maturation of reproductive system and production of sex hormones

OVERVIEW OF JEAN PIAGET'S STAGES OF COGNITIVE DEVELOPMENT

Jean Piaget (1896–1980), the renowned Swiss biologist and psychologist, wrote volumes on his research of child development. Piaget's *theory of cognitive development* states that motor activity involving concrete objects results in the development of mental functioning. For example, as an infant discovers his hand holding a rattle, he begins to recognize a sound that occurs every time he moves the hand holding the rattle. Therefore, reflex activity drops out as repetition produces a result that the infant observes: his activity begins to take on purpose. Eventually, the infant identifies the shaking rattle as a producer of sound. Later, he will realize that he is able to create the sound.

Cognitive refers to the ability to think and reason logically and to understand abstract ideas. Piaget states that, as cognitive development progresses, children gain insights, learn to solve problems, and are able to understand abstract concepts. Children's logic and modes of thinking are, initially, entirely different from those of adults. Piaget believed that cognition progresses through a process of adaptation: assimilation and accommodation. *Assimilation* involves the interpretation of events in terms of existing cognitive knowledge, whereas *accommodation* refers to changing the cognitive knowledge to make sense of the environment. Cognitive development consists of a constant effort to adapt to the environment in terms of assimilation and accommodation. Piaget felt that cognitive development came from the child's interaction with the environment.

Some believe that Piaget's theory is as important to cognitive development as Sigmund Freud's theory is to psychiatry. According to Piaget's theory of cognitive development, each individual needs to make sense of new experiences by relating them to existing understanding. Therefore, every child progresses through each stage of development in the same sequence; however, the timetable may vary from one child to the next. Cognitive development is a continuing process as more of life is experienced.

It should also be remembered that family, culture, personality, and socialization of the sexes may influence individual differences in cognitive development. Recognizing Piaget's developmental periods enables health care professionals to communicate on a level that matches a child's development and understanding. Sharing this information with parents who may be struggling to understand their child may also be beneficial.

Principles applicable to Piaget's theory of cognitive development include the following:

- Children will provide different explanations of reality at different stages of cognitive development.

- Providing activities or situations that engage learners and require adaptation (i.e., assimilation and accommodation) facilitates cognitive development.

- Learning materials and activities should involve the appropriate level of motor or mental operations for a child of a given age; avoid asking children to perform tasks that are beyond their current cognitive capabilities.

- Use teaching methods that actively involve the children's current challenges.

Piaget identified four stages or periods in which children progress in their learning. This table illustrates each of Piaget's cognitive development categories.

TABLE 2 Piaget's Stages of Cognitive Development

Cognition Period and Age Range	Cognitive Activity	Therapeutic Approach and Desired Outcome
Sensorimotor Period: (birth to 2 years)		Provide physical comfort and security to the child and educate the caregiver.
Stage 1 (birth to 1 month)	Sucking and innate reflex activity is paramount. The child does not differentiate between self and other objects.	Provide caregiver education and instruction regarding breast- and bottle-feeding.
Stage 2 (1 to 4 months)	The child begins to make distinctions, repeats simple actions, shows curiosity, and begins hand-to-mouth coordination.	Respond to the "social smile." Hold and support infant so that it feels secure. Infants can roll off the table, so never leave them unattended or take your eyes or hands off them.
Stage 3 (4 to 8 months)	The child experiences increased manipulation and control of objects; repeats rewarding activities and develops eye-to-hand coordination.	The infant recognizes familiar faces and voices, so include parent and/or primary caregiver in procedures where appropriate. Use caution in regard to what is within reach of infants.
Stage 4 (8 to 12 months)	In the period just prior to the first birthday, the child imitates and anticipates events more actively and shows a growing sense of organization of things.	Continue to formulate a positive experience with the infant. Use caution in regard to what is within reach or on the floor—everything goes into the mouth.
Stage 5 (12 to 18 months)	The child explores and experiments more and discovers new ways to get what he/she wants.	Smile when talking to infants of this age. Provide a warm and friendly atmosphere and be consistent. Safety measures must be exercised.
Stage 6 (18 to 24 months)	The child may have imaginary friends and is learning to speak words.	Infant is developing a memory and has some ability to think. Wearing colored uniform tops or jackets or buttons for interest may be helpful. Smile often and "talk" to the infant.
Preoperational Period: (2 to 6 years)	The child does not fully understand quantity, weight, length, and volume. Cannot follow or fully understand reality as it changes; thought is irreversible; cannot understand how something may change and then return to its original condition.	The child focuses attention on only one aspect of a situation. At this age child begins to think symbolically, as demonstrated through language formation, thinking of past and future events, and the ability to pretend and fantasize. Give simple commands and use games and imagery when appropriate.
Concrete Operations: (7 to 11 years)	Child is able to classify objects by category; can focus attention on more than one situation at a time; able to distinguish length, quantity, and weight. Can consider another's point of view; understand that things can be reversed.	Communicate on a level that matches the child's development and understanding. Use praise and rewards to reinforce positive behavior. Allow the child to make decisions when making a wrong decision is not possible. (Should I see how tall you are first or how much you weigh?)
Formal Operations: (12 years to adult)	This stage of adolescence is characterized by hypothetical, logical, and abstract thought processes. Most children can arrive at several possible solutions when given a problem. Long-term goals can be established. Understands symbols, i.e.: political cartoons and algebra. May be idealistic; challenge adult decisions and authority figures.	Help child make sense of new experiences by relating them with existing understanding. Communicate on a level that matches the child's development and understanding. Use praise to reinforce positive behavior.

OVERVIEW OF ABRAHAM MASLOW'S HUMANISTIC PSYCHOLOGY

Abraham Maslow (1908–1970) is considered the founder of humanistic psychology. Maslow was not opposed to other theorists; he simply regarded his work as an extension of modern trends in psychology. He is well known for his **Hierarchy** *of Needs*, which is often used to illustrate motivating forces.

While working with monkeys early in his career, Maslow noticed that some needs took precedence over others. For example, if the monkeys were hungry and thirsty, they would tend to seek water first. You can do without food for weeks, but you can only live without water a few days. If someone had a chokehold on you and you could not breathe, what would be most important? Breathing, of course. Maslow also concluded that sex is less powerful than food, thirst, and air to breathe. No one has ever died from not having sex.

Maslow believed that individuals move back and forth from one need to another, depending upon the circumstances present at the time. He also demonstrated that development continues throughout the life cycle. The following table illustrates Maslow's Hierarchy of Needs.

TABLE 3 Maslow's Hierarchy of Needs

Progression of Need Level	Examples of Specific Needs
Physiologic Needs	oxygen, water, protein, electrolytes, minerals, and vitamins
Safety Needs	safe environment, stability, protection, freedom from fear and anxiety, need for structure, law and order, and limits
Love and Belonging Needs	need to give and receive affection, desires to marry, have a family, be part of a community
Esteem Needs	basic need for a stable, healthy respect for self and others. Desire for achievement, strength, confidence, recognition, prestige, reputation, status, and fame
Self-actualization	achievement of potential—doing what you are truly fitted for

OVERVIEW OF LAWRENCE KOHLBERG'S STAGES OF MORAL DEVELOPMENT

Lawrence Kohlberg (1927–1987) was a psychologist who was born in Bronxville, New York, and served as a professor at Harvard University, where many of his studies on moral development were completed.

Kohlberg developed a theory that moral development is dependent on the thinking and problem-solving stimulated in the child. The theory claims that individuals acquire a sense of justice through a sequence of stages related to cognitive development. The stages closely parallel and are built on Piaget's theory and research.

Progress from one stage to another depends on a person's cognitive development and the opportunity to be exposed to different ideas and experiences. Standards change as society changes. As children grow older, however, discipline given in love seems to be more effective when encouraging moral development than is discipline that is aggressive and controlling.

This table illustrates the six identifiable stages of moral development according to Kohlberg. The stages may be classified into three levels.

TABLE 4 Kohlberg's Stages of Moral Development

Moral Development Level and Orientations	Behavior	Moral Dilemma
Preconventional Level		
Obedience and Punishment Orientation	To do good is to avoid punishment.	Individuals in this level judge the morality of an action by its direct consequences.
Self-Interest Orientation	You be good to me and I'll be good to you.	
Conventional Level		
Conformity Orientation	Child learns to be a "good" boy or girl because there is value in doing so.	Moral behavior is what is accepted and approved by others. Approval becomes more important than reward.
Law-and-Order Orientation	Child learns the importance of obeying the law and social standards.	Law and order as well as fixed rules are recognized, either by religion or social order or both.
Postconventional Level or Principled Level		
Social Contract Orientation	Actions are determined by individual rights or standards, such as the described laws and the U.S. Constitution.	Individuals in this reasoning level think actions are wrong if they violate their ethical principles. Laws may be changed when necessary as long as there is agreement.
Principled Conscience Orientation	Morality becomes individual principles that are logical, comprehensive, and consistent. Justice and equality of human rights, respect, and worthwhile life is recognized. Universal ethical principles are established.	

OVERVIEW OF ERIK ERIKSON'S EIGHT STAGES OF PSYCHOSOCIAL DEVELOPMENT

Erik Erikson (1902–1994) was born in Frankfurt, Germany. His adolescent years were spent wandering through Italy, his young adulthood in Austria working with Freud, and his later life in the United States.

Erikson's psychosocial theory is an approach to personality that extends the Freudian psychosexual theory. Like Freud, Erikson taught that psychological development is a continuous process; each phase or stage is part of a continuum throughout the life cycle. Each developmental stage presents a problem or crisis that the individual must face and master. These **psychosocial crises** are conflicts between a person and society or social institutions. They are the motivating forces behind the individual's behavior. Resolution of each life crisis enhances a person's ability to meet the next crisis and is characterized by hypothetical, logical, and abstract thought processes. The following table illustrates Erikson's eight psychosocial crises.

TABLE 5 Erikson's Stages of Psychosocial Development

Psychosocial Crisis and Age Range	Growth and Development	Therapeutic Approach and Desired Outcome
Trust versus Mistrust (infancy)		Provide physical comfort and security to the child and educate the caregiver.
(birth to 4 weeks)	*Motor Development:* Visual fixation (stares at windows and ceiling); eyes follow bright moving objects; head sags when unsupported; makes crawling movements when prone. *Physical Growth:* Gains 5 to 7 ounces weekly and grows one inch monthly (for 6 months). *Vocalization:* Cries when hungry or uncomfortable, making throaty sounds. Tries to communicate pain or discomfort.	Health care professional should smile and use a pleasant, calm voice when speaking with infant caregivers. Encourage caregivers to verbalize their feelings and concerns and respond to each inquiry. Educate caregiver in understanding that the infant is dependent upon others and how to interpret ways in which the infant makes known those needs. Hold and support the infant so that it feels secure.
(2 months)	*Motor Development:* Eyes are better controlled; can turn body from side to back; can hold head erect, in mid-position. *Physical Growth:* Growth patterns continue; posterior fontanel closed. *Vocalization:* Knows crying will get attention; crying becomes differentiated—for hunger, pain, attention.	Respond to the "social smile." Hold and support the infant so that it feels secure. Remember infants of this age can roll off the table or counter, so never leave them unattended or take your eyes or hands off them. Mobiles over the examination table create a pleasing atmosphere for the infant.

(continues)

TABLE 5 *(continued)*

Psychosocial Crisis and Age Range	Growth and Development	Therapeutic Approach and Desired Outcome
	Socialization: Begins to respond to attention by expressing a "social smile" in response to others.	
(3 months)	*Motor Development*: When prone, infant will rest on forearms and keep head midline; discovers and stares at hands; plays with hands and fingers; able to place hand or object in mouth at will. *Vocalization*: Babbles and coos, laughs aloud; shows pleasure in making sounds; makes initial vowel sounds. *Socialization*: Recognizes parent or primary caregiver.	The infant recognizes familiar faces and voices, so include parent and/or primary caregiver in procedures where appropriate. Use caution in regard to what is within reach of infants, as they are much more active at this stage.
(4 months)	*Motor Development*: Holds head up; can turn body from back to side; recognizes familiar objects; sits with adequate support. *Physical*: Drools (does not know how to swallow saliva); deciduous teeth appear. *Vocalization*: Vocalizes socially (coos when talked to)—very talkative. *Socialization*: Enjoys having people close by; initiates social play by smiling.	Continue to formulate a positive experience with the infant. Use caution in regard to what is within reach or on the floor—everything goes into the mouth.
(6 months)	*Motor Development*: Reaches for objects; grasps objects with whole hand; can hold two objects—one in either hand; can pull self to sitting position; hitches for **locomotion**. *Physical*: Doubles birth weight; continues to gain 3 to 5 ounces weekly and grows one-half inch monthly. *Vocalization*: Vocalizes displeasure as well as several distinguishable syllables; cries easily. *Socialization*: Begins to recognize strangers.	Smile when talking to infants of this age. Provide a warm and friendly atmosphere. Safety measures must be exercised.
(8 months)	*Motor Development*: Bounces and bears some weight when held in	The infant is developing a memory and has some ability to *(continues)*

TABLE 5 *(continued)*		
Psychosocial Crisis and Age Range	**Growth and Development**	**Therapeutic Approach and Desired Outcome**
	standing position; discovers feet; hand-eye coordination is perfected; sits alone; displays exploratory behaviors with food. *Vocalization*: Makes polysyllabic vowel sounds; imitates speech sounds. *Socialization*: Shows fear of strangers and affection for family members.	think. Wearing colored uniform tops or jackets or buttons for interest may be helpful. Smile often and "talk" to the infant.
(10 months)	*Motor Development*: Crawls and creeps; raises self to sitting position; sits alone; preference for use of one hand; manipulates objects; can hold bottle. *Vocalization*: Says one or two words; is able to initiate expression and gestures. *Socialization*: Pays attention to his/her name; plays simple games (pat-a-cake); responds to adult anger (tone of voice).	Involve child in simple games; be aware of the tone of voice used; when child is eating, use care to prevent choking.
(12 months)	*Motor Development*: Stands alone for a moment; walks with help; can sit from standing position without help; can pick up food and transfer to mouth; cooperates in dressing. *Physical*: Triples birth weight; doubles birth length. *Vocalization*: Uses expressive jargon; recognizes meaning of "no-no." *Socialization*: Still egocentric; shows emotions (jealousy, affection, anxiety, and anger); responds to music.	Use praises and rewards to reinforce positive behavior. May play music in examination room. Allow the child to help dress after a procedure.
(12 to 15 months)	*Motor Development*: Walks alone; can release objects at will; tells parent or primary caregiver "I do it"; gets into things; has one-directional thinking—mine, no-no. *Physical*: **Babinski** and **Landau reflexes** disappear. *Vocalization*: Points to indicate wants. *Socialization*: Shares emotions; enjoys being center of attention.	The key element at this stage of development is safety. Use large blocks, stuffed toys that are washable, and cloth books in the reception area and examination room. Do not keep children and parents waiting long; excessive waiting encourages anxiety.

(continues)

TABLE 5 *(continued)*

Psychosocial Crisis and Age Range	Growth and Development	Therapeutic Approach and Desired Outcome
Autonomy versus Shame and Doubt Toddler	The child's energies are directed toward the development of physical skills, including walking, grasping, and rectal sphincter control.	Encourage and praise their physical accomplishments.
(18 to 24 months)	*Motor Development*: Walks up and down stairs; opens doors; turns knobs; uses spoon without spilling; helps undress self; can jump. *Vocalization*: Knows 200 to 300 words; begins to use short sentences. *Socialization*: Obeys simple commands; uses word "mine" constantly; enjoys parallel play (health care professional plays with a puppet while the child also plays with a puppet).	Use simple commands such as "roll over," and "give me the book"; reward acceptable behavior with hugs and stamps on the hand.
(2 to 3 years)	*Motor Development*: Feeds self well; can undress self; walks backwards; begins to use scissors. *Physical*: Has full set of 20 deciduous teeth. *Vocalization*: Knows 900 words. *Socialization*: Negativism grows out of child's sense of developing independence; rituals are important.	Develop a consistent routine for office visits; provide rewards for positive behavior; talk to the child directly as much as possible.
Initiative versus Guilt Preschool age	The child continues to become more assertive and to take more initiative.	Foster initiative to master new tasks.
(3 to 6 years)	*Motor Development*: Dresses self (buttons shirt and ties shoelaces); climbs and jumps well. *Physical*: Growth is relatively slow (gains less than 5 pounds per year and grows 2 to 2 1/2 inches per year). *Socialization*: Talks to imaginary friends; can be given simple explanations as to cause and effect; still needs security of parent's or primary caregiver's presence; initial need to be accepted by others outside the family; strong motivation to measure up.	Give simple explanations and short, simple commands. This age responds well to drawings and play. May give a pretend injection to doll and explain, "This will hurt for a minute. It will help you feel better so you can play."

(continues)

TABLE 5 *(continued)*

Psychosocial Crisis and Age Range	Growth and Development	Therapeutic Approach and Desired Outcome
Industry versus Inferiority Grade school years	The child must deal with demands to learn new skills or risk a sense of inferiority, failure, and incompetence.	Productivity and mastery of skills
(6 to 11 years)	*Motor Development*: Coordination is refined; begins to develop independence; likes to bathe self without assistance. *Physical*: Height increases proportionally to weight gain; begins to lose baby teeth; acquires first molars. *Socialization*: Begins to take responsibility for own actions; begins to accept authority outside the home; uses the telephone; works for acceptance; has to be good at something or feels inferior; no interest in the opposite sex.	Provide encouragement and praise where appropriate. Encourage self-esteem. Explain procedures at the child's level of understanding. Provide choices where appropriate: "Should I check how well you can see first or how well you can hear?"
Identity versus Role Confusion Adolescence	The teenager must achieve a sense of identity in occupation, sex roles, politics, and religion.	Ability to be oneself
(12 to 18 years)	*Motor Development*: Awkward. *Physical*: Females—menstruation begins; axillary and pubic hair becomes coarser and darker; increased development of breasts. Males—grow pubic and facial hair; growth spurts in height; shoulders broaden; voice changes; axillary hair develops; production of **spermatozoa**, **nocturnal emission** may occur. Both males and females—**sebaceous glands** on face, back, and chest become more active. *Socialization*: Increased interest in the opposite sex; concerned with morality, ethics; peer group important; emancipation from family begins.	Peer importance is critical. Provide privacy and remember this group is very modest. They have a fear and concern regarding future changes in body image. Will this procedure or process impact future activity levels?
Intimacy versus Isolation Early Adulthood	The young adult must develop intimate relationships or suffer feelings of isolation.	Capacity for affiliation and love

(continues)

TABLE 5 *(continued)*

Psychosocial Crisis and Age Range	Growth and Development	Therapeutic Approach and Desired Outcome
(19 to 40 years)	This group is interested in the development of a career, searching for a mate, and establishing a home and family. *Physical*: In general, experiencing good health and at their peak. Usually only routine examinations or emergency care for an injury or illness is all that will be needed.	At this stage individuals are self-confident and able to make rational decisions regarding their health care. Provide options and describe the benefits and expectations of good health care.
Generativity versus Stagnation Middle Adulthood (40 to 65 years)	Each adult must find some way to satisfy and support the next generation. This can be the most productive period, as individuals are making and discovering new things. Usually established socioeconomically and do not have to struggle. Begin to think of charity; give back to their parents and community. *Physical*: Health maintenance is important during this stage. Routine examinations and procedures need to be evaluated regularly. A balanced diet and exercise program should be maintained. Attention should be given to stress levels and how to cope with stress in life experiences.	Concern for the succeeding generation. If these clients are not fulfilled, they will feel empty and dissatisfied. They either feel good about the past or they despair. Often they will brag of past accomplishments, reasserting worth. Listen to what they have to say. Provide health care choices when appropriate.
Ego-Integrity versus Despair Late Adulthood (65 to death)	These individuals are beginning to think of retirement or have retired; looking back on their lives and accomplishments. They may be afraid to die or may feel they have not lived life to its fullest. *Physical*: The body or mind or both may begin to fail. Body functions begin to decrease and/or malfunction.	Reflection on and acceptance of one's life; feeling fulfilled. Give these individuals a firm handshake and eye contact; address them by their full name and title; ask their opinion; allow them to make decisions regarding their health care if possible. Do not refer to them using endearing terms such as "dear," "sweetie," "honey."

EXERCISES

Exercise 1

Identify at least five experiences you have had with individuals you could identify as being in one of either Freud's or Erikson's stages of psychosocial development. What actions or evidence helped you make your decision? In a health care setting, how would you communicate therapeutically?

Exercise 2

If you have brothers or sisters or can observe children whose ages are identified in Piaget's period of growth and development, write a brief paper identifying at least five descriptions of activities performed by these children in those periods. Did you observe any children who were performing tasks prior to the age Piaget suggests? Later than suggested? What does this exercise tell you about how you can best communicate with each age group?

Exercise 3

Select two children from a family, day care, or preschool setting. One should be between 4 and 7 years old; the other should be between 7 and 11 years. Perform the following exercises.

Understanding of Length

1. Get two sticks, pieces of yarn, or straws of the same length. Alone with each child, align your sticks, yarn, or straws in front of the child and ask if the items are equal in length. Observe the response. Now move one of your objects a little to the right of the other and ask the child if they are the same length. Observe the response.

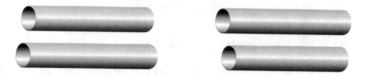

Understanding of Number

2. Using ten pennies, align five pennies in two rows. Again, alone with each child, ask if there are the same number of pennies in each row. Observe the response. Now move one row of pennies further apart and ask if there are the same number of pennies. Observe the response.

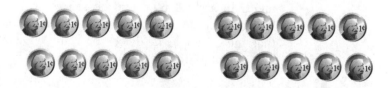

Understanding of Liquid Mass

3. Fill two clear, small, round glasses of the exact same size with the same amount of milk. Alone, ask each child if the liquid in each glass is the same amount. Observe the response. Now pour the milk from one of the glasses into a glass of a taller size and more slender shape. Ask if the glasses now hold the same amount of milk. Observe the response.

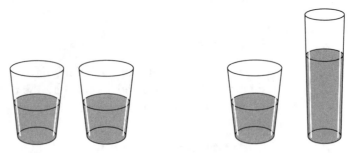

What have you learned from these experiments? Planning the experiments and deciding how to communicate with each child is part of the exercise. Were the children able to understand your instructions? Did they ask for explanations? Was your communication level appropriate for their ages?

What periods of cognitive development most correctly identify your children's reactions?

Exercise 4

A client comes to the dental office in obvious pain and discomfort from a severely abscessed tooth. The client remarks, "I couldn't sleep, I can't eat, and I couldn't go to work today."

Which of Maslow's stages most accurately describes the client?

What action should the health care professional take to assist this client?

Exercise 5

As you reflect upon moral development and the information in this appendix, you have probably been reminded of your own moral development. In a short report to be shared with your instructor, identify the individuals who were influential in your moral development. What is it that these people modeled for you? What other influences have been instrumental in your moral development?

Try to identify *only five* beliefs you have about morality. You may have many more; however, try to determine which five would be the most important. Compare your list of five with others in class. Discuss what might cause these differences. Are the differences related to models? Culture? Religion?

Exercise 6

Consider one of Kohlberg's critic's observation that females view moral issues in a different manner then do males. Do you agree or disagree? Are you able to give examples from your own experience to support your response?

RESOURCES

Frisch, N. C., & Frisch, L. E. (2006). *Psychiatric mental health nursing* (3rd ed.). Clifton Park, NY: Thomson Delmar Learning.

Mandleco, B. L. (2004). *Growth & development handbook: newborn through adolescent.* Clifton Park, NY: Thomson Delmar Learning.

Smith, L. (2007). *A short biography of Jean Piaget.* Retrieved June 18, 2007 from http://www.piaget.org/aboutPiaget.html

Thornton, S. P. (2005). *The Internet encyclopedia of philosophy.* Retrieved December 27, 2005 from http://www.iep.utm.edu/f/freud.htm

APPENDIX

B

DEFENSE MECHANISMS

INTRODUCTION

The term **defense mechanisms** has been defined as behavior that is used to protect the ego from guilt, anxiety, or loss of esteem. Using defense mechanisms is a process the unconscious uses to combat and fight anxiety. It is the body's way of seeking relief or guarding itself from uncomfortable feelings.

An individual wishing to block an emotionally painful experience may, subconsciously or consciously, use a defense mechanism. This enables the individual to put a problem on hold until sufficient time has elapsed to work through the situation and arrive at a solution, or come to terms of acceptance.

The use of defense mechanisms may be healthy or unhealthy. It may be considered an unhealthy approach if the problem is never resolved. Behavior resulting from the use of defense mechanisms may be inappropriate in later developmental stages. An example might be the child who throws a temper tantrum in an effort to get the parents' attention. Then, during early school years, this same child becomes the class clown in order to seek attention from those in authority.

The use of defense mechanisms is difficult to analyze, since it is the motive behind the behavior that characterizes the various mechanisms and gives them their individuality. Some mechanisms may be used to provide time to adjust to and accept a problem, while others may be used to cope with or survive a situation. Some commonly used defense mechanisms are described in Appendix B.

Compensation is consciously or unconsciously overemphasizing a characteristic to compensate for a real or imagined deficiency. For example, the young boy whose physical stature may keep him from being a football star may compensate by achieving an academic award.

Denial is the unconscious refusal to acknowledge painful realities, feelings, or experiences. Denial offers a temporary escape from an unpleasant event. For example, when a laboratory report comes back positive and the client is told, they may express denial by saying, "There must be a mistake!"

Displacement is shifting the emotional element of a situation from a threatening object to a non-threatening one. An example is the client who is very angry with the physician for not explaining a procedure completely. When the client leaves the office, the door is slammed really hard, when in reality, the physician is being "slammed."

Projection is attributing one's own thoughts or impulses to another individual as if they had originated in the other person. Usually negative or unacceptable feelings or urges are projected. From this perspective, every bad choice made is someone else's fault. For example, the drug-dependent to read client who blames someone else because there is no money to pay the rent or buy food.

Rationalization is the mind's way of justifying behavior by offering an explanation other than a truthful response. It is often used to save face or avoid embarrassment. There is usually some grain of truth in the explanation. For example, the client told by the physical therapist to exercise the neck several times a day for five minutes may respond with an excuse such as, "I couldn't do the exercises that often because I had to go to work." The client could have done the exercises seated at a desk.

Regression is an attempt to go back to an earlier stage of development to escape fear, anxiety, or conflict. Toddlers who have been toilet trained for a year or two when a new baby arrives in the household may become anxious or feel displaced and regress to soiling themselves again.

Repression is the unconscious blocking from awareness material that is threatening or painful. It is the mind's way of forgetting or experiencing temporary amnesia until it can cope with an overwhelming circumstance. Clients with post-traumatic stress syndrome may use repression to deal with things too painful to face.

Suppression is the conscious or unconscious attempt to keep threatening material out of consciousness. It is deliberately refusing to acknowledge something that causes mental pain or suffering. An example would be the failure to remember a significant childhood event, such as the death of a grandmother.

Sublimation is redirecting a socially unacceptable impulse into socially acceptable behavior. For example, the artist who expresses sexual impulses in sculpture or paintings is sublimating.

Undoing is canceling out a behavior or trying to make amends. The individual is trying to make up for an inappropriate behavior and the guilty feelings that accompany the act. An abusive person often showers the abused with gifts after the abusive event, hoping to "undo" the unacceptable behavior.

EXERCISES

Exercise 1

Review the list of defense mechanisms. Identify the one you use most often. List three instances when you used it in the last two weeks, and describe the results.

Exercise 2

Enjoy an evening watching your favorite television programs. List the defense mechanisms you observe and describe how these were used and the results of their use.

RESOURCES

Frisch, N. C., & Frisch, L. E. (2006). *Psychiatric mental health nursing* (3rd ed.). Albany, NY: Thomson Delmar Learning.

Lindh, W. W., Pooler, M. S., Tamparo, C. D., & Dahl, B. M. (2006). *Comprehensive medical assisting: administrative and clinical competencies* (3rd ed.). Albany, NY: Thomson Delmar Learning.

Milliken, M. E. (2004). *Understanding human behavior: a guide for health care providers* (7th ed.). Albany, NY: Thomson Delmar Learning.

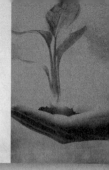

GLOSSARY

Acrophobia Fear of high places.

Acute Having rapid onset, severe symptoms, and a short course.

Adaptive energy This energy influences the body's resistance to stress, is inherited, and varies from one individual to another. The ability of the body to adapt to stressors.

Addiction Physiological or psychological dependence on a substance that is beyond voluntary control.

Agorophobia Fear of public places; usually developes after one or more panic attacks.

Amulets Something worn on the body as a charm against evil.

Anticipatory grief Grief experienced prior to the actual loss.

Anxiety A vague, uneasy feeling of discomfort or dread accompanied by an autonomic response.

Authoritarian Leaders who use a domineering and direct communication style when managing personnel.

Autonomic nervous system The part of the nervous system that controls involuntary bodily functions.

Autonomy versus Shame and Doubt Erikson's psychosocial crisis from 18 to 24 months of age.

Babinski reflex A reflex action of the toes, indicative of abnormalities in the motor control pathways.

Bias A slant toward a particular belief.

Bipolar depression (BPD) Also known as manic-depression and manic-depressive illness. BPD alternates between extreme highs of mania and severe lows of depression.

Child abuse Deliberate harm or injury of child by parent or caretaker.

Chronic Illness with a long duration.

Classical Conditioning A procedure in which a conditioned stimulus, through repeated pairings with an unconditioned stimulus, comes to elicit the conditioned response. (For example, a dog is given food when a bell is rung. The dog's response is to salivate. After repetition, the dog will salivate when the bell is rung, even when it is not given food.)

Claustrophobia Fear of being confined in a small space.

Clichés Patterned responses; trite expressions; empty, meaningless phrases.

Clinical depression Depression with symptoms severe enough to disrupt the client's daily life and requiring medical intervention.

Clustering Grouping of gesutre, facial expressions, and postures into nonverbal statements.

Cognitive The ability to think and reason logically and to understand abstract ideas.

Compensation Consciously or unconsciously overemphasizing a characteristic to compensate for a real or imagined deficiency.

Concrete Operations Piaget's cognition period from 7 to 11 years of age.

Conscience The part of self that judges the self in terms of values and activity; the superego.

Conventional level Kohlberg's theory that moral behavior is what is accepted and approved by others.

Cultural brokering The act of bridging, linking, or mediating between culturally diverse groups or individuals.

Culture A pattern of many concepts, beliefs, values, habits, skills, instruments, and art of a given group of people in a given period.

Defense mechanisms Behavior that protects the psyche from guilt, anxiety or shame.

Denial Unconscious refusal to acknowledge painful realities, feelings, or experiences.

Depression A condition of feeling sadness that may include symptoms such as hopelessness, loss of appetite, sleep disruption, anxiety, low energy, inability to feel pleasure, and thoughts of suicide.

Detoxification A period of time in which to rid the body of the abused substance.

Diagnostic and Statistical Manual (DSM) Published by the American Psychiatric Association. Used by mental health care professionals for a wide range of purposes, including clinical, research, administrative and educational.

Dialect The form of a spoken language peculiar to a region, social group, etc.

Displacement Shifting the emotional element of a situation from a threatening object to a nonthreatening one.

Drug Enforcement Agency Federal agency that identifies and enforces controlled substance regulations.

Dysfunctional grief Grief that is unresolved.

Dysthymic disorder Clients suffer from recurrent or long-lasting depression. These clients almost always seem to have symptoms of a mild form of depression.

Ebonics African American Vernacular English (AAVE), known colloquially as Ebonics, also called Black English.

Ego The psychological force that is in touch with reality and mediates between the id and the superego.

Ego-ideal Corresponds to the child's conceptions of what the parents or primary caregivers consider to be morally good.

Ego-Integrity versus Despair Erikson's psychosocial crisis from 65 years of age to death.

Elder Abuse Deliberate harm or neglect inflicted on someone who is 60 years old or older.

Endogenous depression Type of depression that comes from within and implies there is no discernable cause for the depression.

Endorphins Chemicals in the brain that are responsible for postitive moods.

Erogenous zones Body areas that provide pleasurable sensations.

Ethnic Referring to people grouped according to a common racial, national, tribal, religious, linguistic, or cultural origin.

Ethnocentrism The belief that one's own group or culture is superior to all other groups or cultures.

Eustress Good stress; optimal amount of stress which helps to promote health and growth

Expectations Personal beliefs or mental images of an event or outcome.

Folk medicine Traditional medicine practiced without a scientific understanding of the processes involved, usually handed down to the common people from earlier times.

Four humors The four humors were four fluids that were thought to permeate the body and influence its health. The concept was developed by ancient Greek thinkers.

General Adaptation Syndrome (GAS) The syndrome described by Hans Selye as the total organism's nonspecific response to stress.

Generativity versus Stagnation Erikson's psychosocial crisis from 40 to 65 years of age.

Health Insurance Portability and Accountability Act of 1996 (HIPAA) Government rules, regulations, and procedures resulting from legislation designed to protect the confidentiality of patient information.

Hierarchy Arranged to a specific order or rank; sequential arrangement.

High-context communications Communication style that involves great reliance on body language, reference to objects in the environment, and culturally relevant phraseology to convey an idea. Relies on the listener knowing related events through close association with the speaker or culture.

Holistic medicine Form of alternative medicine that focuses on 1) personal accountability for one's health; 2) the human body's ability to heal itself; and 3) balancing the body, mind, and "spirit" with the environment.

Homeostasis State of balance within the internal environment of the body.

Hospice An interdisciplinary program of palliative care and supportive services that addresses the physical, spiritual, social, and economic needs of terminally ill clients and their families. This care may be provided in the home or a hospice center.

Hypochondriasis Abnormal anxiety and fears regarding one's health.

Id A person's basic animal nature; it is unconscious and amoral.

Identity versus Role Confusion Erikson's psychosocial crisis from 12 to 18 years of age.

Idioms An idiom is an expression whose meaning is not compositional—that is, whose meaning does not follow from the meaning of the individual words of which it is composed.

Industry versus Inferiority Erikson's psychosocial crisis from 6 to 11 years of age.

Initiative versus Guilt Erikson's psychosocial crisis from 3 to 6 years of age.

Instrumental conditioning Learned response through reinforcement. Also known as *operant conditioning*.

Internal milieu Internal environment.

International Classification of Disease (ICD) Standard diagnosis codes used to identify a client's medical problem.

Intimacy versus Isolation Erikson's psychosocial crisis from 19 to 40 years of age.

Intimate partner violence (IPV) Physical, sexual, or psychological/emotional violence directed toward a spouse or former spouse, current or former partner, or current or former dating partner.

Involutional depression Also known as melancholia.

Kinesics Study of the body and its static and dynamic position as a means of communication.

Kosher food Prepared in accordance with Jewish dietary laws.

Landau reflex When an infant is held in the prone position, the entire body forms a convex upward arc.

Leaven A substance used to produce fermentation in dough or a liquid.

Life-altering An illness that affects or limits the quality of life. Some chronic illnesses and most life-threatening illnesses are life-altering illnesses.

Locomotion Ability to move from one place to another; hitch and pull self for movement.

Low-context communication Communication style that utilizes few environmental or cultural idioms to convey an idea or concept. Ideas are spelled out explicitly.

Major depression The most severe category of depression, with more intense or severe symptoms of depression present.

Minor depression A subclinical depression that is less severe and does not meet criteria for major depression diagnosis.

Nocturnal emission Involuntary discharge of semen during sleep.

Nonreciprocal Interchange or performance that is one-sided; respect may not go both ways.

Oedipus Child identifies with and desires sensual satisfaction from the parent of the opposite sex and views the parent of the same sex as a rival.

Operant conditioning Learned response through reinforcement. Also known as *instrumental conditioning.*

Oriental medicine Oriental medicine is really a catchall term for the forms of acupuncture, herbal medicine, massage, and exercise that originated in Asia and are now practiced worldwide. It is the most widely integrated form of energy medicine in Western cultures. Traditionally used for prevention, it has garnered acclaim for successful treatment of a variety of acute and chronic conditions without the adverse side effects found in Western medicine.

Palliative Relieving or alleviating without curing.

Paradigms A set of implied assumptions or beliefs held by an individual or cultural group. As used in this text, the assumptions are based on incorrect information, i.e., "all doctors are men."

Paranoid Ideation The feeling, suspicion or belief that one is being unfairly treated, harassed, or persecuted based on weak circumstantial evidence. Willingness to concede feelings are incorrect when confronted with evidence to the contrary.

Parasympathetic nervous system The craniosacral division of the autonomic nervous system.

Participative Leaders who elicit suggestions from subordinates and encourage open discussion.

Perceptions The images people have in their minds of places, situations, or events. Perceptions may differ from reality.

Pleasure principle Immediate gratification or primitive drives; whatever satisfies an impulse is good and whatever blocks or frustrates it is bad.

Postconventional Level The first level of Kohlberg's theory on moral development. Individuals' ethical principles are guided by consequences.

Postpartum depression A depression that follows childbirth in some mothers.

Preconventional Level Kohlberg's theory that punishment and reward are understood. To do good is to avoid punishment.

Prejudice The process of "prejudging" something, usually in a biased manner.

Preoperational Period Piaget's cognition period from 2 to 6 years of age.

Projection Attributing one's own thoughts or impulses to another individual as if they had originated in the other person.

Psychosocial crises Conflicts between a person and society or social institutions.

Race People who are believed to belong to the same genetic stock.

Racism Racism is a form of discrimination based on race, especially the belief that one race is superior to another. Racism may be expressed individually and consciously; through explicit thoughts, feelings, or acts; or socially and unconsciously, through institutions that promote inequality between races.

Rationalization The mind's way of justifying behavior by offering an explanation that is other than a truthful response.

Reactive depression A state of depression that is precipitated by events in the person's life (to be distinguished from normal grief).

Reality principle That which exists; what is real.

Regionalism Speech or manners representative of a specific geographical location.

Regression An attempt to go back to an earlier stage of development to escape fear, anxiety, or conflict.

Repression Mind's way of forgetting or experiencing temporary amnesia until it can cope with an overwhelming circumstance.

Rituals In organizational aspect of life, used to reinforce the routines and "the way things are done around here."

Seasonal Affective Disorder (SAD) A depression that occurs each year at the same time, usually starting in fall or winter and ending in spring or early summer.

Sebaceous glands Glands that secrete oily or fatty substance.

Self-actualization Fulfilling one's ultimate potential.

Self-awareness Knowing oneself as an individual.

Sensorimotor Period Piaget's cognition period from birth to 2 years of age.

Sodomy Anal intercourse.

Somatic Pertaining to the body; i.e. physiological illness.

Spermatozoa Male sex cell; sperm.

Stalking Repeated behavior causing someone high levels of fear.

Stereotyping The habit of attaching an uncomplimentary or generalized label to a person, race, idea, or the like.

Stress State of mental or emotional strain resulting from physical, physiological, or psychological stressors.

Stressor Stimuli, environmental factors, or life events that result in physiological arousal or stress.

Sublimation Redirecting a socially unacceptable impulse into socially acceptable behavior.

Substance Use Disorder (SUD) Substance abuse and addiction.

Substance-induced mood disorder A type of depression precipitated by the use of prescription drugs.

Superego The moral branch of the personality; the ideal self; strives for perfection.

Suppression Deliberately refusing to acknowledge something that causes mental pain or suffering.

Sympathetic nervous system The thoracolumbar division of the autonomic nervous system.

Trust versus Mistrust Erikson's Psychosocial Crisis from birth to 18 months of age.

Undoing To cancel out a behavior or to try to make amends.

Unipolar disorder A recurrent mood disorder consisting solely of a state of intense sadness, melancholia or despair that has advanced to the point of being disruptive to an individual's social functioning and/or activities of daily living.

Western medicine A term used by to describe allopathic medicine, orthodox medicine, or the way medicine has traditionally been practiced in the United States and Europe. Western medicine utilizes the scientific method and employs pharmaceuticals combined with surgical procedures to combat disease and illness.

INDEX

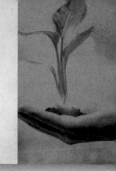